HOW TO FUEL YOUR BODY FOR OPTIMAL PERFORMANCE:
A COMPREHENSIVE GUIDE TO NUTRITION AND EXERCISE FOR PEAK PERFORMANCE

BY
HENRY E. PARKINS

1

COPYRIGHT PAGE

HENRY E. PARKINS

TABLE OF CONTENTS

4

INTRODUCTION

In a world where demands are high and challenges are constant, the quest for peak performance is more than just a pursuit it's a necessity. Whether you're an athlete striving for victory, a professional aiming for career excellence, or simply someone seeking to thrive in everyday life, the fuel you provide your body plays a critical role in achieving your goals.

Welcome to "How to Fuel Your Body for Optimal Performance: A Comprehensive Guide to Nutrition and Exercise for Peak Performance." This book is your roadmap to unlocking the full potential of your body and mind through the power of nutrition and exercise.

In the pursuit of greatness, optimal performance is not just about reaching your peak for a fleeting moment; it's about sustaining that peak and continuously pushing your boundaries. It's about feeling energized, focused, and ready to tackle whatever challenges lie ahead. And at the core of this journey is the synergy between what you eat and how you move.

The pages ahead are dedicated to unraveling the intricacies of nutrition and exercise, offering insights, strategies, and practical advice to help you optimize your performance in every aspect of life. Whether you're an experienced athlete looking to fine-tune your regimen or a newcomer eager to embark on a journey of self-improvement, this book is designed to meet you where you are and guide you toward your aspirations.

Throughout these chapters, you'll discover the fundamental principles of nutrition and exercise, explore the science behind fueling your body for success, and learn how to design personalized plans tailored to your unique needs and goals. From understanding the role of macronutrients and micronutrients to mastering the art of effective workout routines, each section is crafted to empower you with knowledge and actionable steps toward sustainable performance enhancement.

But this book is more than just a collection of guidelines and recommendations it's a testament to the transformative power of intentional living. It's about fostering a mindset of resilience, discipline, and self-discovery as you strive to become the best version of yourself. It's about embracing the journey, embracing the process, and embracing the potential within you to achieve greatness.

As you embark on this enlightening journey through the world of nutrition and exercise, remember that your path to optimal performance is uniquely yours. Along the way, you may encounter obstacles, setbacks, and moments of doubt but with dedication, perseverance, and the right tools at your disposal, you have the power to overcome any challenge and emerge stronger than ever before.

So, whether you're flipping through these pages for guidance, inspiration, or a newfound sense of purpose, know that you hold the key to unlocking your full potential. Your journey toward peak performance starts here let's fuel your body, ignite your passion, and soar to new heights together.

Importance of Optimal Performance in Daily Life and Various Endeavors

In the pursuit of success and fulfillment, optimal performance stands as a cornerstone, guiding individuals toward their aspirations and empowering them to realize their full potential. Whether in the realm of sports, career, academics, or personal relationships, achieving peak performance is not merely a desirable outcome it's a vital component of leading a purposeful and enriching life.

Enhanced Productivity and Efficiency:

Optimal performance equips individuals with the tools and capabilities needed to excel in their endeavors. By fine-tuning their skills, sharpening their focus, and maximizing their energy levels, individuals can enhance their productivity and efficiency, achieving more in less time and with greater precision.

Achievement of Goals and Ambitions:

At the heart of optimal performance lies the pursuit of goals and ambitions. Whether aiming to win a championship, advance in one's career, or accomplish personal milestones, peak performance serves as the catalyst for turning aspirations into reality. By harnessing the power of nutrition and exercise, individuals can propel themselves toward their desired outcomes with clarity, determination, and unwavering commitment.

Physical and Mental Well-Being:

Beyond external achievements, optimal performance encompasses the holistic well-being of individuals, nurturing both their physical and mental health. By prioritizing nutrition and exercise, individuals can cultivate resilience, vitality, and a sense of balance that not only enhances their performance but also promotes longevity and overall quality of life.

11

Resilience in the Face of Challenges:

Inevitably, life presents its fair share of challenges and adversities. However, those who cultivate optimal performance are better equipped to navigate turbulent waters with grace and resilience. By maintaining a strong foundation of physical health and mental fortitude, individuals can weather storms, overcome obstacles, and emerge from setbacks stronger and more resilient than before.

Inspiration and Leadership:

Optimal performance serves as a beacon of inspiration, igniting the potential within individuals and inspiring others to pursue greatness alongside them. Whether as leaders in their respective fields or as mentors to those around them, individuals who embody peak performance have the power to uplift, motivate, and empower others to strive for excellence in their own lives.

Significance of Nutrition and Exercise in Achieving Peak Performance

At the core of peak performance lies the symbiotic relationship between nutrition and exercise a dynamic duo that fuels the body, sharpens the mind, and unlocks the full potential of individuals striving for excellence. Understanding the significance of nutrition and exercise is essential for anyone committed to achieving their peak performance in all aspects of life.

Fueling the Body for Success:

Nutrition serves as the foundation upon which peak performance is built. The foods we consume provide the raw materials necessary for energy production, muscle repair, cognitive function, and overall well-being. By nourishing the body with a balanced diet rich in essential nutrients, individuals can optimize their physical and mental capabilities, ensuring they have the energy and vitality needed to excel in their pursuits.

13

Optimizing Physical Health and Fitness: Exercise is the catalyst that transforms potential into reality, strengthening the body, enhancing endurance, and boosting resilience. Through regular physical activity, individuals can improve cardiovascular health, build lean muscle mass, and increase flexibility and mobility all of which are essential components of peak physical performance. Moreover, exercise stimulates the release of endorphins, neurotransmitters that promote feelings of happiness and well-being, fostering a positive mindset conducive to success.

Enhancing Mental Acuity and Focus: The benefits of nutrition and exercise extend beyond the realm of physical health, profoundly impacting cognitive function and mental clarity. Studies have shown that a nutrient-rich diet and regular exercise can improve concentration, enhance memory retention, and sharpen cognitive skills, allowing individuals to perform at their peak in academic, professional, and creative endeavors. By nourishing the brain with essential nutrients and promoting cerebral blood flow through physical activity, individuals can unlock their full intellectual potential and achieve remarkable feats of mental prowess.

Supporting Recovery and Resilience:

In the pursuit of peak performance, rest and recovery are just as crucial as rigorous training and proper nutrition. Adequate sleep, relaxation techniques, and strategic rest periods allow the body to repair and regenerate, reducing the risk of injury, preventing burnout, and promoting long-term sustainability. By incorporating restorative practices into their routines, individuals can optimize their recovery process, bounce back from setbacks, and cultivate the resilience needed to persevere in the face of adversity.

Promoting Longevity and Quality of Life:

The significance of nutrition and exercise extends far beyond immediate performance gains, impacting the trajectory of individuals' lives and influencing their overall health and well-being. By adopting healthy lifestyle habits early on and consistently prioritizing their physical and mental fitness, individuals can mitigate the risk of chronic diseases, enhance their longevity, and enjoy a higher quality of life well into old age.

Overview

"How to Fuel Your Body for Optimal Performance: A Comprehensive Guide to Nutrition and Exercise for Peak Performance" is a definitive resource designed to empower individuals to unlock their full potential and achieve peak performance in all aspects of life. Grounded in the principles of nutrition, exercise science, and holistic wellness, this book offers a comprehensive roadmap for optimizing physical and mental performance through strategic fueling and intentional movement.

Purpose: The purpose of this book is to demystify the complexities of nutrition and exercise, providing readers with practical insights, evidence-based strategies, and actionable steps to enhance their performance and well-being. Whether you're an athlete striving for victory, a professional aiming for career excellence, or simply someone seeking to thrive in everyday life, this book is your ultimate guide to fueling your body for success.

Structure:

1. Provides an overview of the book's purpose and structure.
2. Sets the stage for understanding the significance of nutrition and exercise in achieving peak performance.

Understanding Optimal Performance:

1. Defines optimal performance and explores its importance in various endeavors.
2. Examines the factors influencing performance and introduces the role of nutrition and exercise.

Foundations of Nutrition for Peak Performance:

1. Covers the basic principles of nutrition, including macronutrients and micronutrients.
2. Emphasizes the importance of hydration and nutrient timing for optimal performance.

Designing Your Optimal Nutrition Plan:

1. Guides readers through the process of assessing individual nutritional needs.
2. Provides practical tips for creating balanced meals, snacks, and fueling strategies.

The Role of Exercise in Performance Optimization:

1. Explores the benefits of regular exercise for physical and mental health.
2. Discusses various types of exercises and their applications for different performance goals.

Integrating Nutrition and Exercise for Peak Performance:

1. Highlights the synergy between nutrition and exercise in enhancing performance.
2. Offers guidance on timing meals and snacks with workout sessions and incorporating supplements effectively.

Overcoming Challenges and Obstacles:

1. Addresses common barriers to maintaining a performance-oriented lifestyle.
2. Provides strategies for overcoming motivational slumps, handling social influences, and navigating setbacks.

Monitoring and Adjusting Your Plan:

1. Emphasizes the importance of self-assessment and feedback in performance optimization.

2. Discusses methods for tracking progress and making adjustments to nutrition and exercise plans.

Achieving Sustainable Long-Term Performance:

1. Encourages consistency, gradual improvements, and resilience in the pursuit of peak performance.
2. Offers strategies for preventing burnout, celebrating achievements, and maintaining motivation.

CHAPTER 1

UNDERSTANDING OPTIMAL PERFORMANCE

At the heart of peak performance lies the pursuit of excellence striving to operate at the highest level of physical, mental, and emotional capacity across various domains of life. Optimal performance encompasses a state of being in which individuals consistently achieve their goals, exceed expectations, and experience a sense of fulfillment and satisfaction in their endeavors.

Definition of Optimal Performance:

Optimal performance is characterized by the ability to consistently deliver one's best performance in any given context, whether it be in sports, academics, career, relationships, or personal pursuits. It goes beyond mere competence or proficiency, encompassing a state of mastery and excellence that transcends limitations and pushes boundaries.

Characteristics of Optimal Performance:

Consistency: Optimal performance is marked by a consistent ability to meet or exceed expectations over time, demonstrating reliability and proficiency in one's chosen pursuits.

Resilience: Individuals who achieve optimal performance possess the resilience to persevere in the face of challenges, setbacks, and adversity, bouncing back stronger and more determined than before.

Adaptability: Optimal performance requires the ability to adapt to changing circumstances, environments, and demands, remaining flexible and open to new approaches and strategies.

Focus and Mindfulness:

Maintaining a high level of focus, concentration, and mindfulness is essential for optimal performance, allowing individuals to channel their energy and attention toward their goals with clarity and purpose.

Balance:

Achieving optimal performance involves striking a balance between dedication to one's pursuits and nurturing other aspects of life, including relationships, health, and well-being.

Factors Influencing Optimal Performance:

Optimal performance is influenced by a multitude of factors, including:

Physical Health and Fitness:

Maintaining a strong foundation of physical health and fitness is essential for optimal performance, providing individuals with the energy, vitality, and resilience needed to excel in their endeavors.

Mental and Emotional Well-Being:

Emotional intelligence, mental resilience, and psychological well-being play crucial roles in achieving optimal performance, enabling individuals to manage stress, overcome obstacles, and maintain a positive mindset.

Nutrition and Hydration: Proper nutrition and hydration are fundamental for supporting optimal performance, providing the body and mind with the essential nutrients, fuel, and hydration needed for sustained energy and focus.

Rest and Recovery: Adequate rest, recovery, and sleep are essential components of optimal performance, allowing the body and mind to repair, regenerate, and recharge for future challenges and endeavors.

Environmental Factors: Environmental factors, including social support, organizational culture, and external stressors, can significantly impact an individual's ability to achieve optimal performance.

Definition and Characteristics of Optimal Performance

Optimal performance represents the pinnacle of human achievement, where individuals consistently operate at their highest potential across various domains of life. Rooted in a commitment to excellence and fueled by a combination of physical, mental, and emotional vitality, optimal performance is characterized by several key attributes:

Definition: Optimal performance is the state in which individuals consistently demonstrate mastery, proficiency, and excellence in their chosen endeavors. It transcends mere competence, reflecting a deep-seated commitment to continuous improvement, innovation, and the pursuit of excellence in all aspects of life.

Characteristics:

a. Consistency: Optimal performers exhibit a remarkable level of consistency in their performance, delivering high-quality

results with precision and reliability. Whether in sports, academics, career, or personal pursuits, they demonstrate a steadfast commitment to excellence in every endeavor.

b. Resilience: Resilience is a hallmark of optimal performance, enabling individuals to navigate challenges, setbacks, and adversity with grace and determination. Optimal performers possess the mental fortitude and emotional resilience to overcome obstacles, adapt to change, and emerge stronger than before.

c. Focus and Mindfulness: Optimal performers maintain a laser-like focus and heightened state of mindfulness, channeling their energy and attention toward their goals with unwavering clarity and purpose. They possess the ability to block out distractions, maintain composure under pressure, and remain fully present in the moment.

d. Adaptability: Adaptability is a key characteristic of optimal performance, allowing individuals to thrive in dynamic

and unpredictable environments. Optimal performers embrace change, remain flexible in their approach, and adapt their strategies to meet evolving circumstances and challenges.

e. Balance: Achieving optimal performance requires a delicate balance between dedication to one's pursuits and nurturing other aspects of life, including relationships, health, and well-being. Optimal performers prioritize self-care, maintain healthy boundaries, and cultivate a sense of harmony and equilibrium in their lives.

f. Growth Mindset: Optimal performers embody a growth mindset, viewing challenges as opportunities for learning and growth rather than insurmountable obstacles. They embrace feedback, seek out new experiences, and continuously strive to expand their knowledge, skills, and capabilities.

Factors Influencing Performance, Including Nutrition and Exercise

Achieving peak performance is a multifaceted endeavor influenced by a myriad of factors spanning physical, mental, emotional, and environmental domains. Understanding and optimizing these factors are essential for individuals striving to excel in their pursuits and unlock their full potential. Among the myriad factors influencing performance, nutrition and exercise play pivotal roles in shaping the body and mind for optimal functioning. Here are the key factors influencing performance, including the critical contributions of nutrition and exercise:

Physical Health and Fitness:

Physical health and fitness serve as the foundation of performance excellence. A strong and resilient body is better equipped to withstand the demands of rigorous training, competition, and everyday challenges.

Factors such as cardiovascular endurance, muscular strength, flexibility, and agility significantly impact an individual's ability to perform at their peak.

Mental Resilience and Emotional Well-being:

Mental resilience and emotional well-being are essential for navigating setbacks, managing stress, and maintaining focus and motivation during challenging times.

Cultivating mindfulness, emotional intelligence, and stress management techniques can enhance an individual's capacity to perform under pressure and overcome adversity.

Nutrition:

Nutrition plays a fundamental role in supporting optimal performance by providing the body with the essential nutrients, energy, and hydration needed for sustained activity and recovery.

Proper nutrition fuels physical performance, promotes muscle repair and growth, enhances cognitive function, and regulates mood and energy levels.

29

Balancing macronutrients (carbohydrates, proteins, fats) and micronutrients (vitamins, minerals) is crucial for meeting the body's nutritional needs and optimizing performance outcomes.

Hydration:

Adequate hydration is critical for maintaining optimal performance levels, as even mild dehydration can impair cognitive function, physical endurance, and thermoregulation.

Hydration needs vary based on factors such as climate, activity level, and individual physiology. Ensuring adequate fluid intake before, during, and after exercise is essential for optimal hydration status.

Sleep and Recovery:

Quality sleep and recovery are indispensable components of peak performance, facilitating physical and mental rejuvenation, muscle repair, and memory consolidation.

Prioritizing sleep hygiene, establishing consistent bedtime routines, and incorporating restorative practices such as meditation, stretching, and massage can enhance recovery and promote overall well-being.

Environmental Factors:

Environmental conditions, including climate, altitude, air quality, and social support networks, can influence performance outcomes and affect an individual's ability to thrive in their chosen pursuits.

Creating supportive environments that foster collaboration, motivation, and accountability can enhance performance and contribute to a positive training and competition experience.

Mental and Physical Aspects of Peak Performance

Achieving peak performance encompasses a delicate balance between the mental and physical dimensions of human capability. The synergy between these aspects is instrumental in unlocking one's full potential and achieving excellence across various domains of life. Understanding and optimizing both the mental and physical aspects of peak performance are essential for individuals striving to reach new heights of achievement. Here's an exploration of the mental and physical dimensions of peak performance:

Mental Aspects:

a. Mindset:

A resilient and growth-oriented mindset is essential for peak performance. Cultivating a positive outlook, embracing challenges as opportunities for growth, and maintaining focus and determination in the face of adversity are key components of a winning mindset.

Techniques such as visualization, goal setting, and positive self-talk can help individuals cultivate a resilient mindset and enhance their capacity for peak performance.

b. Focus and Concentration:

Peak performance requires unwavering focus and concentration on the task at hand. Training the mind to block out distractions, maintain attentional control, and stay present in the moment is crucial for achieving optimal results.

Mindfulness practices, meditation, and attentional training exercises can help individuals sharpen their focus and enhance their ability to perform under pressure.

c. Emotional Regulation:

Emotions play a significant role in performance outcomes, influencing decision-making, motivation, and resilience in the face of challenges.

Developing emotional intelligence, self-awareness, and effective coping strategies can help individuals regulate their emotions, manage stress, and maintain composure during high-pressure situations.

Physical Aspects:

a. Strength and Endurance:

Physical strength and endurance are foundational components of peak performance, providing the capacity to sustain effort over prolonged periods and overcome physical challenges.

Strength training, cardiovascular exercise, and endurance-focused activities such as running, swimming, or cycling can help individuals build muscular strength, cardiovascular fitness, and stamina.

b. Flexibility and Mobility:

Flexibility and mobility are essential for optimal movement patterns, injury prevention, and functional performance in everyday activities and athletic endeavors.

Incorporating flexibility exercises, dynamic stretching routines, and mobility drills into a comprehensive training program can improve joint range of motion, reduce the risk of injury, and enhance overall physical performance.

c. Coordination and Agility:

Coordination, balance, and agility are critical for executing precise movements, maintaining body control, and adapting to changing environmental demands.

Activities that challenge coordination and proprioception, such as agility drills, balance exercises, and sport-specific movements, can improve neuromuscular

coordination and enhance athletic performance.

CHAPTER 2

FOUNDATIONS OF NUTRITION FOR PEAK PERFORMANCE

Nutrition serves as the cornerstone of optimal performance, providing the essential nutrients, energy, and support necessary for peak physical and mental function. In "How to Fuel Your Body for Optimal Performance: A Comprehensive Guide to Nutrition and Exercise for Peak Performance," we delve into the foundational principles of nutrition that form the bedrock of success in achieving your performance goals. Here, we explore the key components of nutrition essential for peak performance:

Macronutrients: Understanding the role of macronutrients carbohydrates, proteins, and fats is fundamental to optimizing performance. Carbohydrates serve as the primary energy source for exercise, while proteins support muscle

repair and growth, and fats provide essential fatty acids and fat-soluble vitamins crucial for overall health and performance.

Micronutrients:

Micronutrients such as vitamins and minerals play a vital role in supporting metabolic processes, immune function, and recovery from exercise. Ensuring adequate intake of micronutrients through a diverse and balanced diet is essential for maintaining optimal health and performance.

Hydration:

Proper hydration is critical for performance, as even mild dehydration can impair physical and cognitive function. Understanding the importance of hydration, monitoring fluid intake, and replenishing electrolytes lost through sweat are essential strategies for optimizing performance and preventing dehydration-related issues.

Nutrient Timing:

Timing meals and snacks strategically around workouts can enhance energy levels, support recovery, and maximize performance gains. Pre- and post-workout nutrition strategies, including carbohydrate and protein intake, play a crucial role in fueling workouts, promoting muscle repair, and optimizing recovery.

Individualized Nutrition:

Recognizing that individual nutrition needs vary based on factors such as age, gender, body composition, activity level, and training goals is key to developing personalized nutrition plans tailored to individual needs. Understanding one's unique nutritional requirements and making adjustments accordingly is essential for optimizing performance and achieving desired outcomes.

Quality and Variety: Emphasizing

the importance of consuming a nutrient-dense diet rich in whole, minimally processed foods is central to supporting optimal health and performance. Prioritizing high-quality sources of carbohydrates, proteins, fats, vitamins, and minerals from a variety of food sources ensures a well-rounded and balanced approach to nutrition.

Mindful Eating: Cultivating mindful eating practices, such as paying attention to hunger and fullness cues, savoring flavors and textures, and practicing gratitude for food, fosters a positive relationship with food and promotes mindful food choices that support overall health and well-being.

Sustainable Habits: Building sustainable nutrition habits that align with long-term health and performance goals is essential for maintaining consistency and adherence to healthy eating patterns. Prioritizing sustainability, flexibility, and enjoyment in food choices contributes to long-term success and overall well-being.

Basic Principles of Nutrition

In "How to Fuel Your Body for Optimal Performance: A Comprehensive Guide to Nutrition and Exercise for Peak Performance," understanding the basic principles of nutrition lays the groundwork for achieving peak physical and mental performance. Here are the fundamental principles of nutrition that form the foundation of optimal performance:

Balanced Diet: A balanced diet includes a variety of nutrient-dense foods from all food groups, including fruits, vegetables, whole grains, lean proteins, and healthy fats. Aim to consume a diverse array of foods to ensure adequate intake of essential nutrients, vitamins, and minerals necessary for overall health and performance.

Macronutrients: Macronutrients—carbohydrates, proteins, and fats—provide the energy and building blocks necessary for optimal function. Carbohydrates serve as the primary energy source, proteins support muscle repair and growth, and fats provide essential fatty acids and aid in nutrient absorption.

Micronutrients: Micronutrients such as vitamins and minerals are essential for various metabolic processes, immune function, and overall well-being. Ensure adequate intake of micronutrients through a balanced diet rich in fruits, vegetables,

whole grains, lean proteins, and dairy or dairy alternatives.

Hydration:

Hydration is crucial for optimal performance, as even mild dehydration can impair physical and cognitive function. Drink water regularly throughout the day and pay attention to thirst cues during exercise to maintain proper hydration levels.

Nutrient Timing:

Timing meals and snacks strategically around workouts can optimize energy levels, support recovery, and enhance performance. Prioritize pre- and post-workout nutrition to fuel workouts, replenish glycogen stores, and promote muscle repair and recovery.

Portion Control: Practicing portion control helps regulate calorie intake and maintain a healthy weight. Pay attention to portion sizes and be mindful of hunger and fullness cues to prevent overeating and promote satiety.

Mindful Eating:

Mindful eating involves being present and attentive to the eating experience, including hunger and fullness cues, flavor sensations, and emotional triggers. Practice mindful eating by savoring each bite, eating slowly, and listening to your body's signals.

Quality Over Quantity: Prioritize high-quality, nutrient-dense foods over processed and refined options. Choose whole, minimally processed foods whenever possible to maximize nutrient intake and support overall health and performance.

Individualized Nutrition: Recognize that individual nutrition needs vary based on factors such as age, gender, body composition, activity level, and training goals. Tailor your nutrition plan to meet your specific needs and preferences, and make adjustments as necessary to optimize performance and well-being.

Consistency: Consistency is key to long-term success in nutrition and performance. Establish healthy eating habits and stick to them consistently, making small, sustainable changes over

time to support your goals and maintain progress.

Macronutrients: Carbohydrates, Proteins, and Fats

In "How to Fuel Your Body for Optimal Performance: A Comprehensive Guide to Nutrition and Exercise for Peak Performance," understanding macronutrients carbohydrates, proteins, and fats is essential for maximizing energy, supporting muscle growth and repair, and optimizing overall performance. Let's explore each macronutrient and its role in fueling your body for peak performance:

Carbohydrates:

Role: Carbohydrates serve as the primary energy source for the body, especially during high-intensity exercise and endurance activities. They provide readily available fuel for muscles and the central nervous system.

Sources: Carbohydrates are found in a variety of foods, including grains (such as rice, pasta, and bread), fruits, vegetables, legumes, and dairy products.

Types: Carbohydrates can be categorized into simple carbohydrates (sugars) and complex carbohydrates (starches and fibers). Aim to prioritize complex carbohydrates for sustained energy and overall health.

Timing: Consuming carbohydrates before exercise helps fuel workouts and maintain blood glucose levels. After exercise, carbohydrates aid in glycogen replenishment and muscle recovery.

Proteins:

Role: Proteins are essential for muscle repair, growth, and maintenance. They also play a role in hormone synthesis, enzyme function, and immune support.

Sources: Protein-rich foods include lean meats, poultry, fish, eggs, dairy products, legumes, tofu, tempeh, nuts, and seeds.

Amino Acids: Proteins are composed of amino acids, which are the building blocks of muscle tissue. Essential amino acids must be obtained through diet, as the body cannot produce them independently.

mine

Fats:

Role

Sources: Healthy fat sources include avocados, nuts, seeds, olive oil, fatty fish (such as salmon and mackerel), and plant-based oils.

Types: Fats can be categorized into saturated fats, unsaturated fats (monounsaturated and polyunsaturated), and trans fats. Focus on consuming unsaturated fats, which are heart-healthy and support overall well-being.

Micronutrients: Vitamins and Minerals

In "How to Fuel Your Body for Optimal Performance: A Comprehensive Guide to Nutrition and Exercise for Peak Performance," understanding micronutrients vitamins and minerals is paramount for supporting metabolic processes, immune function, and overall well-being. Let's explore the importance of vitamins and minerals and their role in fueling your body for peak performance:

Vitamins:

Role: Vitamins are essential organic compounds that play key roles in various physiological processes, including energy metabolism, immune function, and tissue repair. They act as cofactors for enzymes and help regulate gene expression.

Sources: Vitamins are found in a wide range of foods, including fruits, vegetables, whole grains, lean proteins, dairy products, and fortified foods.

Types: Vitamins are classified into two categories: fat-soluble vitamins (A, D, E, and K) and water-soluble vitamins (B vitamins and vitamin C). Fat-soluble vitamins are stored in the body's fat tissues, while water-soluble vitamins are excreted through urine and require regular replenishment.

Functions: Each vitamin has specific functions and benefits for health and performance. For example, vitamin D supports bone health and immune function, vitamin C acts as an antioxidant and aids in collagen synthesis, and vitamin B12 is involved in energy metabolism and red blood cell production.

Minerals:

Role: Minerals are inorganic elements that serve as essential cofactors for enzymatic reactions, electrolyte balance, and structural components of tissues and bones. They play critical roles in muscle contraction, nerve transmission, and fluid balance.

Sources: Minerals are found in a variety of foods, including fruits, vegetables, whole grains, lean meats, dairy products, nuts, seeds, and legumes.

Types: Minerals are classified into two categories: macrominerals (required in larger amounts) and trace minerals (required in smaller amounts). Macrominerals include calcium, magnesium, phosphorus, sodium, potassium, and chloride, while trace

47

minerals include iron, zinc, copper, selenium, iodine, and chromium.

Functions: Each mineral serves specific functions in the body, such as calcium and phosphorus for bone health, iron for oxygen transport and energy production, and potassium for muscle function and blood pressure regulation.

Importance of Hydration for Performance

In "How to Fuel Your Body for Optimal Performance: A Comprehensive Guide to Nutrition and Exercise for Peak Performance," understanding the importance of hydration is paramount for maximizing physical and mental performance. Hydration plays a critical role in maintaining fluid balance, regulating body temperature, and supporting various physiological functions essential for peak performance. Let's explore why hydration is key for performance optimization:

Optimal Fluid Balance:

Hydration is essential for maintaining optimal fluid balance in the body. Adequate

48

hydration ensures that cells, tissues, and organs receive the necessary fluids to function efficiently. Maintaining fluid balance is particularly crucial during exercise when fluid losses through sweat increase.

Regulation of Body Temperature: Hydration plays a vital role in regulating body temperature, especially during exercise and physical activity. Sweating is the body's natural mechanism for cooling down and dissipating heat. Proper hydration helps replenish fluids lost through sweat and prevents dehydration, which can lead to overheating and impaired performance.

Energy Production and Nutrient Transport: Hydration supports energy production and nutrient transport throughout the body. Water is involved in various metabolic processes, including the breakdown of carbohydrates, proteins, and fats for energy. Adequate hydration ensures efficient nutrient delivery to cells and tissues, supporting

optimal performance during exercise and daily activities.

Cognitive Function and Mental Clarity:

Proper hydration is essential for maintaining cognitive function, focus, and mental clarity. Even mild dehydration can impair concentration, memory, and decision-making abilities, negatively impacting performance in both physical and cognitive tasks. Staying hydrated helps sustain mental acuity and sharpness, enhancing overall performance.

Muscle Function and Recovery:

Hydration plays a crucial role in supporting muscle function, endurance, and recovery. Dehydration can lead to muscle cramps, fatigue, and decreased exercise performance. Proper hydration helps maintain muscle hydration and electrolyte balance, optimizing muscle function and facilitating faster recovery after exercise.

Prevention of Heat-Related Illnesses:

Adequate hydration helps

prevent heat-related illnesses such as heat exhaustion and heatstroke, which can occur during intense physical activity, especially in hot and humid environments. Proper fluid intake helps regulate body temperature and reduces the risk of heat-related injuries and illnesses.

Optimized Cardiovascular Function: Hydration supports cardiovascular function by maintaining blood volume and circulation. Proper fluid balance ensures adequate blood flow to muscles and organs, optimizing oxygen delivery and nutrient transport during exercise. Optimal hydration also helps prevent cardiovascular strain and enhances cardiovascular efficiency during physical activity.

In summary, hydration is a fundamental aspect of performance optimization, supporting fluid balance, temperature regulation, energy production, cognitive function, muscle function, and overall well-being. By prioritizing hydration and maintaining proper fluid intake before, during, and after exercise, individuals can enhance their physical and mental performance, maximize endurance, and achieve peak performance in their respective endeavors.

CHAPTER 3

DESIGNING YOUR OPTIMAL NUTRITION PLAN

Creating a nutrition plan tailored to your individual needs and goals is a crucial step in fueling your body for optimal performance. Whether you're an athlete striving for peak physical condition, a professional aiming for cognitive sharpness, or someone seeking overall well-being, a well-designed nutrition plan can enhance your energy levels, support recovery, and optimize your overall performance. Here's how to design your optimal nutrition plan:

Assess Your Nutritional Needs:

Begin by assessing your unique nutritional requirements based on factors such as age, gender, activity level, metabolic rate, and specific performance goals.

Consider consulting with a registered dietitian or nutritionist to conduct a comprehensive assessment and receive personalized recommendations based on your individual needs and preferences.

Determine Your Macronutrient Ratios:

Macronutrients carbohydrates, proteins, and fats serve as the building blocks of your nutrition plan and play distinct roles in fueling your body for optimal performance.

Determine the appropriate macronutrient ratios based on your goals, activity level, and metabolic profile. For example, athletes engaged in intense training may require higher carbohydrate and protein intake to support energy production and muscle repair.

Emphasize Whole, Nutrient-Dense Foods:

Prioritize whole, nutrient-dense foods that provide a rich source of vitamins, minerals, antioxidants, and phytonutrients essential for optimal health and performance.

Include a variety of colorful fruits and vegetables, lean proteins, whole grains, healthy fats, and low-fat dairy or dairy alternatives in your daily meals and snacks.

Focus on Timing and Distribution:

Pay attention to the timing and distribution of your meals and snacks throughout the day to optimize energy levels, support recovery, and maintain stable blood sugar levels.

Aim for balanced meals and snacks that include a combination of carbohydrates, proteins, and fats to provide sustained energy and prevent energy crashes.

Consider Pre- and Post-Workout Nutrition:

Pre- and post-workout nutrition plays a crucial role in fueling your workouts, enhancing performance, and supporting recovery.

Consume a balanced meal or snack containing carbohydrates and protein 1-3 hours before exercise to fuel your workout and optimize glycogen stores.

After exercise, replenish lost fluids and electrolytes, and consume a combination of carbohydrates and protein to facilitate muscle recovery and repair.

Stay Hydrated:

Hydration is essential for optimal performance, cognitive function, and overall health. Aim to maintain adequate hydration levels by drinking water throughout the day, especially during periods of increased physical activity or high temperatures.

Monitor your hydration status by paying attention to thirst cues, urine color, and sweat rates, and adjust your fluid intake accordingly.

Address Dietary Restrictions and Preferences:

Consider any dietary restrictions, allergies, or food intolerances you may have when designing your nutrition plan.

Explore alternative food options and creative recipes that align with your dietary preferences and restrictions while still providing the necessary nutrients to support your performance goals.

Monitor and Adjust as Needed:

Regularly monitor your progress, energy levels, performance outcomes, and overall well-being to assess the effectiveness of your nutrition plan.

Be flexible and willing to adjust your nutrition plan based on feedback from your body, performance metrics, and changes in your goals or lifestyle.

Assessing Individual Nutritional Needs

Before embarking on any nutrition plan, it's essential to assess your individual nutritional needs to ensure that your dietary choices align with your goals, lifestyle, and unique physiological requirements. By understanding your body's specific needs, you can tailor your nutrition plan to optimize performance, support recovery, and enhance overall well-being. Here's how to assess your individual nutritional needs:

Conduct a Comprehensive Health Assessment:

Begin by conducting a comprehensive health assessment to evaluate your current health status, medical history, and any existing health conditions or concerns.

Consider factors such as age, gender, weight, height, body composition, metabolic rate, and activity level when assessing your nutritional needs.

Determine Your Baseline Nutrient Requirements:

Determine your baseline nutrient requirements based on established dietary guidelines, recommended daily allowances (RDAs), and dietary reference intakes (DRIs) for key nutrients.

Identify the specific nutrient needs for macronutrients (carbohydrates, proteins, fats) and micronutrients (vitamins, minerals, antioxidants) based on your age, gender, and activity level.

Assess Energy Needs and Expenditure:

Estimate your daily energy needs and expenditure based on your basal metabolic rate (BMR), physical activity level, and any additional energy requirements for growth, recovery, or weight management goals.

Use online calculators, metabolic equations, or consult with a registered dietitian to determine your personalized energy needs.

Consider Performance Goals and Activity Level:

Consider your performance goals, training regimen, and activity level when assessing your nutritional needs.

Individuals engaged in intense physical activity or training may require higher calorie and nutrient intake to support energy expenditure, muscle repair, and recovery.

Evaluate Dietary Preferences and Restrictions:

Take into account your dietary preferences, cultural influences, and lifestyle factors when assessing your nutritional needs.

Identify any dietary restrictions, allergies, intolerances, or ethical considerations that may impact your food choices and nutrient intake.

Monitor Nutrient Intake and Food Choices:

Keep a food diary or use mobile apps to track your nutrient intake, food choices, portion sizes, and eating patterns over time.

Evaluate your nutrient intake against recommended dietary guidelines and adjust your food choices as needed to ensure adequate intake of essential nutrients.

Assess Hydration Status:

Assess your hydration status by monitoring fluid intake, urine output, and signs of dehydration such as thirst, dry mouth, and dark-colored urine.

Aim to consume adequate fluids throughout the day to maintain optimal hydration levels, especially during periods of increased physical activity or exposure to hot temperatures.

Seek Professional Guidance if Needed:

If you're unsure about how to assess your individual nutritional needs or interpret dietary guidelines, consider seeking guidance from a registered dietitian or nutrition professional.

A qualified nutrition expert can provide personalized recommendations, dietary counseling, and practical strategies to help you optimize your nutrition plan for peak performance.

Creating Balanced Meals and Snacks

Balanced meals and snacks are essential components of a nutrition plan designed to fuel your body for optimal performance. By incorporating a variety of nutrient-dense foods into your daily eating routine, you can provide your body with the energy, essential nutrients, and hydration needed to support your performance goals, enhance recovery, and promote overall well-being. Here's how to create balanced meals and snacks that optimize your nutrition for peak performance:

Include a Variety of Macronutrients:

Aim to include a balance of carbohydrates, proteins, and fats in each meal and snack to provide your body with a diverse array of nutrients and energy sources.

Carbohydrates serve as the primary fuel source for high-intensity activities and cognitive function, while proteins support muscle repair and growth, and fats provide sustained energy and support hormone production.

Prioritize Whole, Nutrient-Dense Foods:

Choose whole, minimally processed foods that are rich in vitamins, minerals, antioxidants, and fiber to maximize nutrient intake and support overall health.

Include a variety of colorful fruits and vegetables, lean proteins such as poultry, fish, tofu, legumes, and whole grains such as quinoa, brown rice, and oats in your meals and snacks.

Opt for Complex Carbohydrates:

Choose complex carbohydrates such as whole grains, fruits, vegetables, and legumes over refined carbohydrates and sugary snacks to provide sustained energy and support stable blood sugar levels.

Incorporate sources of fiber-rich carbohydrates, such as leafy greens, sweet potatoes, berries, and beans, to promote satiety and digestive health.

Include Lean Proteins:

Incorporate lean sources of protein into your meals and snacks to support muscle repair, recovery, and growth.

Choose lean cuts of poultry, fish, eggs, tofu, tempeh, Greek yogurt, cottage cheese, and legumes as sources of high-quality protein to complement your meals and snacks.

Incorporate Healthy Fats:

Include sources of healthy fats, such as avocados, nuts, seeds, olive oil, and fatty fish like salmon and trout, to provide essential fatty acids and support brain function, hormone production, and satiety.

Use moderation when incorporating fats into your meals and snacks, as they are calorie-dense and can contribute to overall energy intake.

Pay Attention to Portion Sizes:

Be mindful of portion sizes and aim to create balanced meals and snacks that provide the appropriate amount of calories and nutrients to support your energy needs and performance goals.

Use visual cues such as the palm of your hand or a deck of cards to estimate appropriate portion sizes for proteins, carbohydrates, and fats.

Hydrate Throughout the Day:

Stay hydrated by drinking water throughout the day and incorporating hydrating foods such as fruits, vegetables, and soups into your meals and snacks.

Monitor your fluid intake and aim to drink adequate water before, during, and after exercise to maintain optimal hydration levels and support performance and recovery.

Plan Ahead and Prepare:

Plan ahead and prepare balanced meals and snacks in advance to ensure that nutritious options are readily available when hunger strikes.

Batch cook grains, proteins, and vegetables, and store them in portioned containers for easy grab-and-go meals and snacks throughout the week.

Addressing Dietary Restrictions and Preferences

Navigating dietary restrictions and preferences is an important aspect of optimizing nutrition for peak performance. Whether due to allergies, intolerances, ethical considerations, cultural practices, or personal preferences, understanding how to accommodate individual dietary needs is essential for achieving optimal health and performance. Here's how to address dietary restrictions and preferences effectively:

Identify Dietary Restrictions and Allergies:

Begin by identifying any dietary restrictions, allergies, or intolerances that may impact food choices and nutrient intake.

Keep a record of specific foods or ingredients that trigger allergic reactions or digestive discomfort, and avoid them when planning meals and snacks.

Seek Alternative Food Options:

Explore alternative food options and substitutes that align with dietary restrictions and preferences.

Look for allergy-friendly, gluten-free, dairy-free, or vegan alternatives to common ingredients, and incorporate them into recipes and meal plans as needed.

Read Food Labels and Ingredient Lists:

Practice diligent label reading to identify potential allergens or ingredients that may not align with dietary restrictions.

Familiarize yourself with common food additives, preservatives, and hidden sources of allergens to make informed food choices.

Experiment with Plant-Based Proteins:

Incorporate plant-based protein sources such as tofu, tempeh, legumes, lentils, quinoa, and hemp seeds into your meals and snacks to meet protein needs while accommodating vegetarian or vegan preferences.

Experiment with different cooking methods and flavor profiles to enhance the taste and texture of plant-based protein sources.

Customize Meals and Recipes:

Customize meals and recipes to accommodate individual dietary preferences and flavor preferences.

Experiment with ingredient substitutions, seasoning blends, and cooking techniques to create flavorful and satisfying dishes that meet your nutritional needs and culinary preferences.

Optimize Nutrient Intake:

Focus on optimizing nutrient intake by choosing nutrient-dense foods that align with dietary restrictions and preferences.

Prioritize whole, minimally processed foods such as fruits, vegetables, whole grains, lean proteins, and healthy fats to maximize nutrient density and support overall health and performance.

Incorporate Diversity and Variety:

Embrace diversity and variety in your diet by incorporating a wide range of foods, flavors, and cuisines that reflect cultural diversity and personal preferences.

Explore international cuisines, ethnic foods, and traditional dishes to expand your culinary repertoire and keep meals interesting and enjoyable.

Communicate and Advocate for Your Needs:

Communicate your dietary restrictions and preferences to friends, family members, colleagues, and food service providers to ensure that your needs are respected and accommodated.

Advocate for yourself by asking questions, requesting ingredient information, and seeking out alternative options when dining out or attending social gatherings.

Consult with a Registered Dietitian:

If you're unsure how to navigate dietary restrictions or need personalized guidance, consider consulting with a registered dietitian or nutrition professional.

Pre- and Post-Workout Nutrition Strategies

Optimizing pre- and post-workout nutrition is essential for fueling your body, maximizing performance, and supporting recovery. By strategically timing nutrient intake around exercise sessions, you can enhance energy levels, promote muscle repair and growth, and optimize overall performance. Here are pre- and post-workout nutrition strategies to fuel your body for optimal performance:

Pre-Workout Nutrition:

a. Timing: Consume a balanced meal or snack containing carbohydrates, proteins, and fats 1-3 hours before your workout to fuel your body and optimize performance.

b. Carbohydrates: Choose easily digestible carbohydrates that provide a quick source of energy, such as fruits, whole grains, or a small serving of low-fiber cereal or toast.

c. Proteins: Include a moderate amount of lean protein to support muscle repair

70

and growth, such as Greek yogurt, cottage cheese, eggs, or a protein shake.

d. *Hydration:* Ensure adequate hydration by drinking water or a sports drink before your workout to prevent dehydration and support optimal performance.

e. Avoid heavy or high-fat meals that may cause digestive discomfort during exercise.

During Exercise:

a. Hydration: Stay hydrated by sipping water or a sports drink throughout your workout, especially during prolonged or intense exercise sessions.

b. *Consider consuming* easily digestible carbohydrate snacks, such as energy gels, chews, or sports drinks, for sustained energy and electrolyte replenishment during longer workouts.

Post-Workout Nutrition:

a. Timing: Consume a combination of carbohydrates and protein within 30-60 minutes after your workout to replenish glycogen stores, promote muscle recovery, and optimize recovery.

b. *Carbohydrates:* Choose fast-digesting carbohydrates to replenish glycogen stores and restore energy levels, such as fruits, whole grains, or sports drinks.

c. *Proteins:* Include a source of high-quality protein to support muscle repair and synthesis, such as lean meats, poultry, fish, tofu, beans, or a protein shake.

d. *Hydration:* Rehydrate by drinking water or a sports drink to replace fluids lost during exercise and support recovery.

e. *Consider adding a small amount* of healthy fats, such as nuts, seeds, or avocado, to your post-workout meal or snack to enhance satiety and support nutrient absorption.

Nutrient Timing and Personalization:

a. Experiment with different pre- and post-workout nutrition strategies to determine what works best for your body and performance goals.

b. **Consider** individual factors such as exercise intensity, duration, timing, and personal preferences when designing your pre- and post-workout nutrition plan.

c. *Listen to your* body's hunger and satiety cues, and adjust your nutrient intake and timing accordingly to optimize performance and recovery.

Supplement Considerations:

a. *Some athletes* may benefit from specific supplements to enhance performance, support recovery, or address nutrient deficiencies. Consult with a healthcare professional or registered dietitian before adding supplements to your regimen.

b. *Common supplements used* for pre- and post-workout nutrition include

73

branched-chain amino acids (BCAAs), creatine, beta-alanine, caffeine, and electrolyte replacements.

CHAPTER 4

THE ROLE OF EXERCISE IN PERFORMANCE OPTIMIZATION

Exercise is a cornerstone of performance optimization, playing a pivotal role in enhancing physical, mental, and emotional well-being to unlock your full potential. Whether you're an athlete striving for peak performance, a fitness enthusiast pursuing personal goals, or an individual seeking to improve overall health and vitality, integrating regular exercise into your routine can yield profound benefits. Here's an exploration of the multifaceted role of exercise in performance optimization:

Physical Fitness and Strength:

Exercise is instrumental in developing physical fitness, strength, and endurance, which are essential components of peak performance across various domains.

Resistance training, cardiovascular exercise, and functional movement patterns help build muscular strength, cardiovascular endurance, and overall physical resilience.

Enhanced Energy Levels and Vitality:

Regular exercise boosts energy levels, improves circulation, and enhances oxygen delivery to tissues, resulting in increased vitality and stamina.

Engaging in physical activity stimulates the release of endorphins, neurotransmitters, and hormones that promote feelings of well-being, mood elevation, and stress reduction.

Improved Cognitive Function and Mental Sharpness:

Exercise has profound effects on cognitive function and mental acuity, enhancing memory, focus, attention, and executive functioning.

Aerobic exercise, in particular, promotes neurogenesis, synaptic plasticity, and the release of brain-derived neurotrophic factor (BDNF), which supports brain health and cognitive resilience.

Stress Reduction and Mood Enhancement:

Physical activity serves as a powerful antidote to stress, anxiety, and depression, promoting relaxation, emotional balance, and psychological well-being.

Exercise triggers the release of neurotransmitters such as serotonin, dopamine, and norepinephrine, which regulate mood, promote feelings of happiness, and mitigate symptoms of mood disorders.

Enhanced Recovery and Injury Prevention:

Incorporating appropriate exercise modalities into your routine can facilitate recovery, reduce muscle soreness, and enhance tissue repair following intense physical activity or training.

Implementing proper warm-up, cool-down, and flexibility exercises can improve joint mobility, reduce the risk of injury, and promote musculoskeletal health and resilience.

Performance Adaptations and Skill Development:

Consistent training and practice lead to performance adaptations and skill development, enabling individuals to refine technique, optimize movement patterns, and achieve mastery in their chosen pursuits.

Deliberate practice, feedback, and progressive overload are key principles that drive skill acquisition, motor learning, and performance improvement over time.

Longevity and Quality of Life:

Regular exercise is associated with improved longevity, reduced risk of chronic diseases, and enhanced quality of life across the lifespan.

Engaging in physical activity promotes cardiovascular health, metabolic health,

78

bone density, immune function, and overall resilience to age-related decline and disease.

Benefits of Regular Exercise for Physical and Mental Health

Regular exercise is a cornerstone of optimal health and vitality, offering a myriad of benefits for both physical and mental well-being. From enhancing cardiovascular fitness to improving mood and cognitive function, integrating regular exercise into your lifestyle can have transformative effects on your overall health and performance. Here are the key benefits of regular exercise for physical and mental health:

Improved Cardiovascular Health:

Regular exercise strengthens the heart muscle, improves blood circulation, and enhances cardiovascular fitness.

Engaging in aerobic activities such as walking, running, cycling, and swimming can lower blood pressure, reduce LDL cholesterol levels, and decrease the risk of heart disease and stroke.

Enhanced Muscular Strength and Endurance:

Exercise stimulates muscle growth, improves muscle tone, and enhances muscular strength and endurance.

Resistance training, bodyweight exercises, and functional movements help build lean muscle mass, increase metabolism, and support overall physical resilience.

Weight Management and Metabolic Health:

Regular physical activity helps maintain a healthy body weight, regulate metabolism, and prevent obesity and metabolic disorders.

Exercise increases energy expenditure, promotes fat loss, and improves insulin sensitivity, leading to better blood sugar control and reduced risk of type 2 diabetes.

Bone Health and Density:

Weight-bearing exercises such as walking, jogging, dancing, and weightlifting promote bone health and density, reducing the risk of osteoporosis and fractures.

Exercise stimulates bone remodeling, strengthens bone tissue, and enhances calcium absorption, leading to stronger, more resilient bones.

Enhanced Flexibility and Joint Health:

Incorporating flexibility exercises, stretching routines, and mobility drills into your exercise regimen improves joint range of motion, reduces stiffness, and prevents musculoskeletal injuries.

Stretching and mobility work promote better posture, reduce muscle tension, and enhance overall functional movement patterns.

Stress Reduction and Mood Enhancement:

Exercise is a powerful stress management tool that reduces cortisol levels, promotes relaxation, and enhances mood and emotional well-being.

Physical activity stimulates the release of endorphins, neurotransmitters, and brain-derived neurotrophic factor (BDNF), which alleviate symptoms of anxiety, depression, and stress.

Improved Cognitive Function and Brain Health:

Regular exercise enhances cognitive function, memory, attention, and executive functioning by promoting neuroplasticity and brain connectivity.

Aerobic exercise increases blood flow to the brain, stimulates the growth of new neurons, and enhances synaptic plasticity, leading to improved learning, mental clarity, and cognitive performance.

Better Sleep Quality and Recovery:

Engaging in regular exercise improves sleep quality, promotes relaxation, and regulates circadian rhythms, leading to deeper, more restorative sleep.

Adequate rest and recovery are essential for muscle repair, recovery from exercise-induced fatigue, and overall physical and mental rejuvenation.

Types of Exercises for Different Performance Goals

Tailoring your exercise routine to specific performance goals is essential for maximizing results and achieving peak performance. Whether you're aiming to improve strength, endurance, agility, or flexibility, incorporating a variety of exercise modalities can help you optimize your training regimen and reach your desired outcomes. Here are types of exercises for different performance goals:

Strength Training:

Goal: Increase muscular strength, power, and lean muscle mass.

Exercises: Focus on compound movements that target major muscle groups, such as squats, deadlifts, bench presses, overhead presses, rows, and pull-ups.

Techniques: Use moderate to heavy weights, perform multiple sets and repetitions (e.g., 8-12 reps per set), and incorporate progressive overload to challenge muscles and stimulate growth.

Endurance Training:

Goal: Improve cardiovascular endurance, stamina, and aerobic capacity.

Exercises: Include aerobic activities such as running, cycling, swimming, rowing, and hiking that elevate heart rate and sustain activity over extended periods.

Techniques: Incorporate steady-state cardio sessions, interval training, and long-duration workouts to build endurance, improve oxygen utilization, and increase tolerance to fatigue.

Flexibility and Mobility:

Goal: Enhance joint range of motion, flexibility, and functional movement patterns.

Exercises: Focus on dynamic stretches, static stretches, and mobility drills that target major muscle groups and joints.

Techniques: Perform yoga, Pilates, tai chi, or mobility exercises such as hip circles, shoulder rotations, and trunk twists to improve flexibility, reduce stiffness, and prevent injury.

Power and Explosiveness:

Goal: Develop explosive strength, speed, and power for athletic performance.

Exercises: Incorporate plyometric exercises such as box jumps, jump squats, medicine ball throws, and explosive sprints that involve rapid muscle contractions and maximal effort.

Techniques: Emphasize quick, explosive movements with minimal ground contact time to improve reactive strength, coordination, and neuromuscular efficiency.

Agility and Coordination:

Goal: Enhance agility, balance, coordination, and proprioception.

Exercises: Include agility drills, ladder drills, cone drills, and sport-specific movement patterns that challenge agility, footwork, and multidirectional speed.

Techniques: Focus on precise movements, quick changes of direction, and reaction time to improve agility, spatial awareness, and sport-specific skills.

Core Stability and Balance:

Goal: Strengthen the core muscles, improve stability, and enhance balance and postural control.

Exercises: Incorporate core exercises such as planks, bridges, Russian twists, stability ball exercises, and unilateral exercises that engage the core and stabilizing muscles.

Techniques: Perform exercises that challenge balance, proprioception, and

86

core activation to improve functional stability and reduce the risk of injury.

Mental Conditioning and Mindfulness:

Goal: Enhance mental resilience, focus, concentration, and stress management.

Exercises: Practice mindfulness meditation, deep breathing exercises, visualization techniques, and mental imagery to cultivate mental toughness and emotional regulation.

Techniques: Incorporate mindfulness practices into your daily routine, set intentions for training sessions, and develop mental strategies to overcome challenges and setbacks.

Incorporating Recovery and Rest into Exercise Routines

While exercise is crucial for optimizing performance and achieving peak physical condition, equally important is the incorporation of recovery and rest into your exercise routine. Proper recovery strategies allow your body to repair, regenerate, and adapt to the stresses of exercise, leading to enhanced recovery, reduced risk of injury, and improved overall performance. Here are key principles for incorporating recovery and rest into exercise routines:

Prioritize Sleep Quality and Quantity:

Aim for 7-9 hours of quality sleep per night to support physical and mental recovery, hormone regulation, and cellular repair processes.

Create a conducive sleep environment by maintaining a consistent sleep schedule, limiting exposure to screens before bedtime, and optimizing sleep hygiene practices.

Implement Active Recovery Strategies:

Incorporate active recovery sessions such as low-intensity cardio, yoga, stretching, or foam rolling to promote blood flow, reduce muscle soreness, and enhance flexibility.

Engage in light physical activity on rest days to facilitate recovery without overstressing the body.

Listen to Your Body:

Pay attention to signs of fatigue, soreness, and overtraining, and adjust your exercise intensity, volume, and frequency accordingly.

Practice intuitive training by allowing for flexibility in your exercise routine based on how your body feels and responds to training stimuli.

Hydrate and Replenish Electrolytes:

Stay hydrated by drinking water throughout the day and replenishing electrolytes lost through sweat during exercise.

Consider consuming electrolyte-rich beverages or snacks, such as coconut water or sports drinks, to maintain electrolyte balance and support hydration.

Incorporate Periodization and Deload Weeks:

Implement periodization principles by varying training intensity, volume, and frequency over time to prevent plateaus, optimize performance, and minimize the risk of overtraining.

Schedule deload weeks or recovery phases into your training program to allow for active recovery, reduced training volume, and mental rejuvenation.

Practice Stress Management Techniques:

Incorporate stress management techniques such as meditation, deep breathing exercises, mindfulness practices, and relaxation techniques to reduce stress levels and promote overall well-being.

Manage external stressors effectively by prioritizing time for relaxation, hobbies, and activities that bring joy and fulfillment.

Nutrition and Hydration for Recovery:

Consume nutrient-dense foods rich in carbohydrates, proteins, and healthy fats to support muscle repair, glycogen replenishment, and recovery.

Optimize post-workout nutrition by consuming a balanced meal or snack containing carbohydrates and proteins to facilitate muscle recovery and replenish energy stores.

Allow for Adequate Rest Days:

Schedule regular rest days into your exercise routine to allow for complete physical and mental recovery.

Use rest days as an opportunity to engage in leisure activities, spend time outdoors, and prioritize self-care practices that promote relaxation and rejuvenation.

CHAPTER 5

INTEGRATING NUTRITION AND EXERCISE FOR PEAK PERFORMANCE

Achieving peak performance requires a holistic approach that integrates nutrition and exercise strategies to optimize fueling, recovery, and overall well-being. By synergistically aligning dietary choices with training regimens, individuals can enhance energy levels, support muscle repair, and maximize physical and mental performance. Here's a comprehensive guide to integrating nutrition and exercise for peak performance:

Understanding Energy Balance:

Energy balance is the foundation of peak performance, where the calories consumed through nutrition match the energy expended during exercise and daily activities.

Balance energy intake from carbohydrates, proteins, and fats with energy expenditure to maintain optimal body composition and support performance goals.

Pre-Workout Nutrition Strategies:

Consume a balanced meal or snack containing carbohydrates, proteins, and fats 1-3 hours before exercise to fuel performance and enhance endurance.

Choose easily digestible carbohydrate sources such as fruits, whole grains, or energy bars for quick energy release.

Include lean proteins such as chicken, fish, or tofu to support muscle repair and growth, along with healthy fats for sustained energy.

Post-Workout Nutrition Strategies:

Refuel within 30-60 minutes after exercise with a combination of carbohydrates and proteins to replenish glycogen stores, support muscle recovery, and promote adaptation.

Opt for fast-digesting carbohydrates like fruits, rice, or potatoes to restore energy levels, coupled with lean proteins such as whey protein, eggs, or Greek yogurt to stimulate muscle protein synthesis.

Hydrate adequately with water or electrolyte-rich beverages to replace fluids lost through sweat and support recovery.

Macronutrient Timing and Distribution:

Distribute macronutrients strategically throughout the day to support energy levels, muscle repair, and metabolic function.

Consume carbohydrates before and after workouts to fuel activity and replenish glycogen stores.

Include protein-rich foods with each meal and snack to support muscle protein synthesis and satiety.

Incorporate healthy fats into meals to support hormone production, brain function, and nutrient absorption.

Hydration and Electrolyte Balance:

Maintain optimal hydration levels by drinking water throughout the day and during exercise to support thermoregulation, nutrient transport, and cellular function.

Consume electrolyte-rich foods and beverages, such as sports drinks, fruits, and vegetables, to replenish electrolytes lost through sweat and prevent dehydration.

Individualized Nutrition Plans:

Tailor nutrition plans to individual needs, preferences, and performance goals, considering factors such as age, gender, body composition, activity level, and training intensity.

Experiment with different nutrient ratios, meal timing strategies, and food combinations to optimize performance, recovery, and overall well-being.

Periodization and Adjustments:

Periodize nutrition and exercise regimens to align with training cycles, competition schedules, and performance objectives.

Adjust nutrient intake and exercise intensity based on training demands, recovery status, and progress toward goals.

Mindful Eating and Enjoyment:

Practice mindful eating by tuning into hunger cues, savoring flavors, and fostering a positive relationship with food and body.

Enjoy a variety of nutrient-dense foods, flavors, and cuisines to meet nutritional needs while enhancing satisfaction and adherence to dietary guidelines.

Choosing Optimal Foods for Pre- and Post-Workout Fueling

Fueling your body with the right foods before and after workouts is essential for optimizing performance, supporting muscle recovery, and enhancing overall well-being. By selecting nutrient-dense foods that provide the right balance of carbohydrates, proteins, and fats, you can maximize energy levels, promote muscle repair, and facilitate recovery. Here's a comprehensive guide to choosing optimal foods for pre- and post-workout fueling:

Pre-Workout Fueling:

Before your workout, focus on consuming a balanced meal or snack that provides sustained energy and supports optimal performance. Aim to eat 1-3 hours before exercise to allow for digestion and absorption. Choose foods that are easily digestible and rich in carbohydrates to fuel your workout, along with a moderate amount of protein to support muscle repair and growth. Here are some optimal pre-workout food options:

a. *Complex Carbohydrates:* -

Whole grains: Brown rice, quinoa, oats, whole grain bread, or pasta provide a steady source of energy and help maintain stable blood sugar levels. - Fruits: Bananas, apples, berries, and oranges are rich in natural sugars and provide quick-digesting carbohydrates for immediate energy. - Sweet potatoes: Rich in complex carbohydrates and vitamins, sweet potatoes offer sustained energy and support glycogen replenishment.

b. *Lean Proteins:* - Greek yogurt: High

in protein and low in fat, Greek yogurt provides essential amino acids for muscle repair and recovery. - Chicken or turkey: Lean sources of poultry are rich in protein and amino acids, which support muscle maintenance and growth. - Tofu or tempeh: Plant-based protein sources like tofu and tempeh offer complete proteins and are suitable options for vegetarians and vegans.

c. Healthy Fats: - Avocado: Loaded with healthy fats and fiber, avocados provide sustained energy and support nutrient absorption. - Nuts and seeds: Almonds, walnuts, chia seeds, and flaxseeds are rich in omega-3 fatty acids and provide lasting satiety.

d. Hydration: - Water: Stay hydrated by drinking water before your workout to prevent dehydration and support optimal performance. - Coconut water: Rich in electrolytes, coconut water helps replenish fluids and maintain hydration levels during exercise.

Post-Workout Recovery:

After your workout, refuel your body with a combination of carbohydrates and proteins to replenish glycogen stores, repair muscle tissue, and promote recovery. Consume a post-workout meal or snack within 30-60 minutes after exercise to maximize nutrient absorption and enhance recovery. Focus on nutrient-dense foods that provide a blend of carbohydrates, proteins, and fluids to support muscle repair and replenish energy stores. Here are some optimal post-workout food options:

a. Fast-Digesting Carbohydrates:

- Rice cakes: Low in fat and easily digestible, rice cakes provide quick-digesting carbohydrates for glycogen replenishment. - Fruit smoothie: Blend fruits like bananas, berries, and spinach with Greek yogurt or protein powder for a refreshing post-workout snack. - White potatoes: Boiled or mashed white potatoes offer fast-digesting carbohydrates and support glycogen replenishment.

b. Lean Proteins:

- Whey protein shake: Easily digestible and rich in essential amino acids, whey protein shakes are ideal for post-workout recovery and muscle repair. - Grilled salmon or tuna: Rich in omega-3 fatty acids and high-quality protein, fish promotes muscle recovery and reduces inflammation. - Cottage cheese: Low in fat and high in protein, cottage cheese is a convenient post-workout snack that supports muscle repair and growth.

c. Recovery Beverages: - Chocolate milk: With an optimal ratio of carbohydrates to protein, chocolate milk provides essential nutrients for recovery and hydration. - Electrolyte sports drinks: Choose electrolyte-rich beverages to replenish fluids, restore electrolyte balance, and prevent dehydration after intense exercise.

Supplements: Benefits, Risks, and Considerations

Supplements can play a role in supporting nutritional needs and optimizing performance, but it's important to understand their benefits, risks, and considerations. While some supplements may offer advantages in specific circumstances, others may pose risks or have limited evidence supporting their efficacy. Here's a comprehensive guide to supplements for optimizing performance and well-being:

Benefits of Supplements:

a. Fill Nutritional Gaps: Supplements can help fill nutritional gaps in the diet, especially for individuals with dietary restrictions, deficiencies, or increased nutrient needs.

b. Enhance Performance: Certain supplements, such as creatine, caffeine, and beta-alanine, have been shown to enhance athletic performance, increase strength, and delay fatigue.

c. Support Recovery: Supplements like protein powders, branched-chain amino acids (BCAAs), and tart cherry juice may support muscle recovery, reduce soreness, and improve post-exercise recovery.

d. Convenience: Supplements offer a convenient way to consume specific nutrients, especially for individuals with busy lifestyles or limited access to whole foods.

Risks and Considerations:

a. Lack of Regulation: The supplement industry is not closely regulated, and products may vary widely in quality, purity, and safety. It's essential to choose supplements from reputable brands that undergo third-party testing for quality and purity.

b. *Potential Side Effects*: Some supplements may cause adverse effects or interactions with medications. It's important to research potential side effects and consult with a healthcare professional before starting any new supplement regimen.

c. *Cost:* Supplements can be expensive, and the cost can add up over time, especially if multiple supplements are used. Prioritize whole foods as the primary source of nutrients whenever possible.

d. *Limited Evidence:* While some supplements have robust scientific evidence supporting their efficacy, others have limited or conflicting evidence. Be cautious of supplements that make exaggerated claims or lack scientific support.

e. *Individual Variation:* The effectiveness of supplements can vary depending on individual factors such as genetics, diet, lifestyle, and training status.

What works for one person may not work the same way for another.

Choosing Supplements Wisely:

a. *Do Your Research:* Prioritize supplements that have been extensively researched and shown to be safe and effective for their intended purpose.

b. *Consult with a Professional:* Before starting any new supplement regimen, consult with a registered dietitian, sports nutritionist, or healthcare provider to assess your individual needs and potential risks.

c. *Consider Whole Foods First:* Whenever possible, prioritize whole foods as the primary source of nutrients. Whole foods offer a variety of nutrients, fiber, and phytochemicals that may not be present in supplements.

d. *Read Labels Carefully:* Pay attention to ingredient lists, dosage recommendations, and potential allergens when selecting supplements. Choose products with minimal additives, fillers, and artificial ingredients.

e. *Monitor Effects:* Keep track of how supplements affect your body and performance. If you experience any adverse effects or discomfort, discontinue use and consult with a healthcare professional.

CHAPTER 6

OVERCOMING CHALLENGES AND OBSTACLES

Embarking on the journey towards optimal performance and well-being through nutrition and exercise is not without its challenges and obstacles. However, by adopting a resilient mindset, strategic planning, and effective problem-solving strategies, you can overcome barriers and navigate setbacks along the way. Here are some key strategies for overcoming challenges and obstacles on your path to peak performance:

Set Realistic Goals:

Define clear, achievable goals that are specific, measurable, and realistic. Break larger goals into smaller, actionable steps to maintain motivation and momentum.

Cultivate Resilience:

Embrace challenges as opportunities for growth and learning. Develop resilience by reframing setbacks as temporary obstacles and focusing on solutions rather than dwelling on problems.

Prioritize Consistency:

Consistency is key to long-term success. Establish sustainable habits and routines that prioritize regular exercise, nutritious eating, adequate sleep, and stress management.

Stay Flexible and Adaptive:

Be willing to adapt and adjust your approach as circumstances change. Remain flexible in your strategies and open to new ideas, methods, and approaches to overcome challenges.

Seek Support and Accountability:

Surround yourself with a supportive network of friends, family, coaches, mentors, or peers who can offer encouragement, guidance, and accountability.

Share your goals and challenges with others, and seek feedback, advice, and assistance when needed.

Practice Self-Compassion:

Be kind to yourself and acknowledge that setbacks and obstacles are a natural part of the journey. Practice self-compassion and treat yourself with the same kindness and understanding you would offer to others.

Focus on Progress, Not Perfection:

Celebrate small victories and milestones along the way. Recognize that progress is incremental and nonlinear, and focus on continuous improvement rather than perfection.

Learn from Setbacks:

View setbacks as valuable learning experiences that provide insights into areas for growth and development. Reflect on challenges, identify lessons learned, and use them to inform future decisions and actions.

Develop Problem-Solving Skills:

Approach challenges with a problem-solving mindset. Break down complex problems into smaller, manageable tasks, and brainstorm creative solutions to overcome obstacles.

Practice Patience and Persistence:

Understand that meaningful change takes time and effort. Practice patience and perseverance, and trust in the process as you work towards your goals.

Common Barriers to Maintaining a Performance-Oriented Lifestyle

Despite our best intentions, maintaining a performance-oriented lifestyle centered around nutrition and exercise can be challenging due to various barriers that we encounter. Recognizing these barriers and developing strategies to overcome them is essential for sustaining long-term success and achieving optimal performance. Here are some common barriers individuals may face:

Time Constraints:

Busy schedules, work commitments, family responsibilities, and social obligations can make it difficult to prioritize exercise and meal planning.

Solution: Schedule workouts and meal prep sessions into your calendar as non-negotiable appointments. Prioritize activities that align with your performance goals and delegate tasks when possible.

Lack of Motivation:

Low motivation, boredom with routine, and feelings of burnout can derail efforts to maintain a performance-oriented lifestyle.

Solution: Set compelling goals, find activities you enjoy, and vary your workouts to keep them engaging and challenging. Surround yourself with supportive individuals and seek inspiration from role models and success stories.

Financial Constraints:

The cost of gym memberships, specialized equipment, organic foods, and supplements can present financial barriers to maintaining a performance-oriented lifestyle.

Solution: Explore cost-effective exercise options such as outdoor activities, bodyweight workouts, and online resources. Budget and prioritize spending on essentials that support your health and performance goals.

Lack of Knowledge:

Limited knowledge about nutrition, exercise techniques, and performance optimization strategies can hinder progress and lead to confusion.

Solution: Educate yourself through reliable sources, books, courses, and reputable websites. Consult with certified professionals such as registered dietitians, personal trainers, and sports coaches for personalized guidance and advice.

Social Influences:

Peer pressure, social norms, and cultural practices may not always align with a performance-oriented lifestyle, leading to temptation and resistance.

Solution: Surround yourself with like-minded individuals who support your goals and share similar values. Communicate your priorities and boundaries with friends and family, and seek out social environments that promote health and well-being.

Emotional Eating and Stress:

Emotional eating, stress, anxiety, and emotional triggers can lead to unhealthy eating habits, overeating, and emotional barriers to consistent exercise.

Solution: Practice stress management techniques such as mindfulness, meditation, deep breathing, and journaling. Develop healthier coping mechanisms for managing emotions and seek professional support if needed.

Physical Limitations and Injuries:

Chronic health conditions, injuries, physical limitations, and disabilities may pose challenges to maintaining a performance-oriented lifestyle.

Solution: Work with healthcare professionals, physical therapists, and rehabilitation specialists to develop safe and effective exercise programs tailored to your needs and capabilities. Focus on activities that improve mobility, function, and overall well-being.

Lack of Supportive Environment:

Unsupportive social environments, negative influences, and lack of encouragement from peers or family members can undermine efforts to maintain a performance-oriented lifestyle.

Solution: Advocate for your needs, communicate your goals, and seek out supportive communities, groups, and networks online or in-person. Surround yourself with individuals who uplift and empower you to thrive.

Strategies for Overcoming Motivational Slumps and Setbacks

Motivational slumps and setbacks are common challenges that individuals encounter on their journey towards optimal performance and well-being. During these times, maintaining momentum and staying committed to nutrition and exercise goals can feel especially challenging. However, with the right strategies and mindset, you can overcome motivational slumps and setbacks and regain your focus and enthusiasm. Here are some effective strategies to help you navigate through these periods:

Reflect on Your Why:

Reconnect with your underlying reasons for pursuing a performance-oriented lifestyle. Reflect on your goals, values, and aspirations, and remind yourself of the benefits and rewards of staying committed to your journey.

Set Realistic Expectations:

Acknowledge that setbacks and fluctuations in motivation are natural and part of the process. Set realistic expectations for yourself, and understand that progress may not always be linear. Celebrate small victories and milestones along the way.

Break Goals into Smaller Steps:

Break down larger goals into smaller, manageable steps that feel less overwhelming. Focus on taking one step at a time, and celebrate each small achievement as you progress towards your larger objectives.

Find Meaningful Rewards:

Identify meaningful rewards or incentives that can help motivate you during challenging times. Whether it's treating yourself to a relaxing massage, enjoying a favorite activity, or indulging in a healthy reward, find ways to celebrate your progress and accomplishments.

Cultivate a Positive Mindset:

Cultivate a positive and resilient mindset by reframing challenges as opportunities for growth and learning. Embrace setbacks as valuable lessons that can strengthen your resilience and determination.

Practice Self-Compassion:

Be kind to yourself during periods of low motivation and setbacks. Recognize that it's okay to have off days and that self-criticism only undermines your progress. Practice self-compassion and treat yourself with the same kindness and understanding you would offer to a friend.

Mix Up Your Routine:

Inject variety into your nutrition and exercise routines to keep things fresh and engaging. Explore new recipes, try different workout formats, and experiment with alternative forms of physical activity to reignite your enthusiasm.

Create a Supportive Environment:

Surround yourself with supportive individuals who uplift and encourage you on your journey. Share your struggles and successes with friends, family members, or fellow enthusiasts who understand and support your goals.

Visualize Success:

Use visualization techniques to imagine yourself achieving your goals and experiencing the benefits of optimal performance. Visualize the positive outcomes of your efforts, and let these visions inspire and motivate you to keep moving forward.

Seek Accountability:

Find an accountability partner, coach, or mentor who can help keep you motivated and on track. Share your goals and progress with someone who can offer guidance, support, and encouragement when needed.

Focus on the Process:

Shift your focus from outcomes to the process of growth and self-improvement. Embrace the journey of self-discovery and personal development, and trust in the process as you work towards your goals.

Handling Social and Environmental Influences on Dietary and Exercise Choices

Social and environmental influences play significant roles in shaping our dietary and exercise habits. From peer pressure to cultural norms, various factors can impact our choices related to nutrition and physical activity. Learning to navigate these influences effectively is essential for maintaining a performance-oriented lifestyle. Here are strategies for handling social and environmental influences on dietary and exercise choices:

Awareness and Mindfulness:

Be mindful of the social and environmental cues that influence your dietary and

118

exercise decisions. Pay attention to how your surroundings, social circles, and cultural norms impact your choices.

Set Clear Boundaries:

Establish clear boundaries and priorities for your health and well-being. Communicate your goals and intentions with friends, family members, and colleagues, and assertively advocate for your needs.

Surround Yourself with Supportive Individuals:

Surround yourself with individuals who support and encourage your performance-oriented lifestyle. Seek out like-minded friends, workout partners, and mentors who share similar values and goals.

Educate and Inform Others:

Educate your social circle about the importance of nutrition and exercise for optimal performance and overall health. Share evidence-based information and resources to help dispel myths and misconceptions.

Lead by Example:

Lead by example by demonstrating healthy eating habits and consistent exercise routines. Show others how prioritizing nutrition and physical activity contributes to vitality, energy, and overall well-being.

Plan Ahead for Social Gatherings:

Plan ahead for social gatherings and events where food and drink choices may not align with your goals. Offer to bring a healthy dish or snack to share, or eat a balanced meal before attending to avoid overindulging.

Practice Assertiveness and Self-Advocacy:

Practice assertiveness and self-advocacy skills to assert your needs and preferences in social and environmental settings. Politely decline offerings that do not align with your dietary or exercise goals, and offer alternatives when possible.

Find Alternative Social Activities:

Explore alternative social activities that prioritize health and well-being, such as group fitness classes, outdoor adventures, or active hobbies. Surround yourself with individuals who enjoy activities that support your performance goals.

Adapt to Social and Environmental Changes:

Stay flexible and adaptable in response to social and environmental changes. Anticipate challenges and setbacks, and develop coping strategies to navigate them effectively.

Create Supportive Environments:

Create supportive environments at home, work, and in your community that foster healthy behaviors and positive choices. Advocate for wellness initiatives and resources that promote nutrition and exercise as integral components of a healthy lifestyle.

Seek Professional Guidance:

Seek guidance from registered dietitians, personal trainers, and health coaches who can provide personalized support and guidance tailored to your individual needs and goals.

CHAPTER 7

MONITORING AND ADJUSTING YOUR PLAN

Monitoring and adjusting your nutrition and exercise plan is essential for optimizing performance, achieving goals, and maintaining long-term success. By regularly assessing your progress, identifying areas for improvement, and making necessary adjustments, you can fine-tune your approach and stay on track towards peak performance. Here's a comprehensive guide to monitoring and adjusting your plan:

Set Clear Goals:

Define clear, specific, and measurable goals for your nutrition and exercise plan. Whether it's improving endurance, building strength, or optimizing body composition, establish goals that align with your aspirations and priorities.

Track Your Progress:

Monitor your progress regularly using objective measures such as body weight, body composition, performance metrics, and subjective indicators like energy levels, mood, and recovery. Keep a journal or use tracking apps to record your data consistently.

Assess Nutritional Intake:

Evaluate your nutritional intake by keeping track of your food choices, portion sizes, macronutrient balance, and overall calorie intake. Use food journals, meal planning tools, or nutrition apps to monitor your dietary habits and identify areas for improvement.

Evaluate Exercise Performance:

Assess your exercise performance by tracking workout intensity, duration, frequency, and progression over time. Keep records of strength gains, cardiovascular endurance, flexibility, and other relevant fitness metrics to gauge improvement and identify plateaus.

Listen to Your Body:

Pay attention to signals from your body, such as hunger, satiety, fatigue, soreness, and recovery. Tune in to how different foods, exercises, and training modalities affect your physical and mental well-being.

Identify Patterns and Trends:

Look for patterns and trends in your data to identify areas of success and areas for improvement. Notice recurring themes, correlations, and discrepancies that can inform your decision-making process.

Seek Feedback:

Seek feedback from qualified professionals such as registered dietitians, sports nutritionists, personal trainers, and healthcare providers. Share your progress, challenges, and goals, and leverage their expertise to guide your adjustments.

Be Flexible and Adaptive:

Stay flexible and adaptive in your approach to nutrition and exercise. Be willing to experiment with different strategies, techniques, and protocols to find what works best for your body and lifestyle.

Make Gradual Adjustments:

Make gradual adjustments to your nutrition and exercise plan based on your assessment findings. Focus on making small, sustainable changes rather than drastic overhauls, and monitor how these adjustments impact your progress.

Celebrate Successes and Learn from Setbacks:

Celebrate your successes and achievements along the way, no matter how small. Acknowledge the progress you've made and the obstacles you've overcome. Use setbacks as opportunities for learning and growth, and adjust your plan accordingly.

Stay Committed and Consistent:

Stay committed to your goals and trust in the process of continuous improvement. Stay consistent with your efforts, even when progress seems slow or obstacles arise. Remember that consistency is key to long-term success.

The Importance of Self-Assessment and Feedback

Self-assessment and feedback are crucial components of optimizing performance in nutrition and exercise. They serve as valuable tools for individuals to evaluate progress, identify areas for improvement, and make informed decisions regarding their health and well-being. Here's why self-assessment and feedback are essential in the journey towards peak performance:

Evaluation of Progress:

Self-assessment allows individuals to objectively evaluate their progress towards their nutrition and exercise goals. By tracking metrics such as weight, body composition, performance, and overall well-being, individuals can gauge the effectiveness of their strategies and make adjustments as needed.

Identification of Strengths and Weaknesses:

Through self-assessment, individuals can identify their strengths and weaknesses in their nutrition and exercise routines. By recognizing areas of proficiency and areas that require improvement, individuals can develop targeted approaches to enhance their performance and overcome challenges.

Awareness of Habits and Behaviors:

Self-assessment promotes self-awareness of habits and behaviors related to nutrition and exercise. By reflecting on dietary choices, exercise patterns, and lifestyle factors, individuals can gain insight into how their behaviors impact their health outcomes and overall performance.

Accountability and Responsibility:

Self-assessment fosters accountability and responsibility for one's health and well-being. By taking ownership of their progress and outcomes, individuals become empowered to make proactive choices that align with their goals and values.

Adaptation and Flexibility:

Feedback from self-assessment enables individuals to adapt and adjust their nutrition and exercise strategies based on evolving needs and circumstances. By remaining flexible and responsive to changes, individuals can optimize their approach to better support their performance goals.

Continuous Improvement:

Self-assessment promotes a culture of continuous improvement and lifelong learning. By embracing feedback and seeking opportunities for growth, individuals can strive for excellence and pursue ongoing refinement in their nutrition and exercise practices.

Empowerment and Autonomy:

Engaging in self-assessment empowers individuals to take an active role in their health and well-being. By developing a deeper understanding of their bodies and needs, individuals can make informed decisions and exercise greater autonomy over their nutrition and exercise choices.

Alignment with Personal Values:

Self-assessment allows individuals to align their nutrition and exercise practices with their personal values and priorities. By reflecting on what matters most to them, individuals can establish meaningful goals and pursue paths that resonate with their unique aspirations and aspirations.

Tracking Progress and Performance Metrics

Tracking progress and performance metrics is an essential aspect of optimizing nutrition and exercise for peak performance. By monitoring key indicators of progress, individuals can assess the effectiveness of their strategies, identify areas for improvement, and stay motivated on their journey towards optimal performance. Here's a comprehensive guide to tracking progress and performance metrics:

Establish Clear Goals:

Begin by establishing clear, specific, and measurable goals related to nutrition, exercise, and overall performance. Define your objectives in terms of weight management, body composition, strength, endurance, flexibility, and other relevant metrics.

Choose Relevant Metrics:

Identify metrics that are relevant to your goals and priorities. Consider metrics such as body weight, body fat percentage, muscle mass, circumference measurements, cardiovascular fitness, strength levels, exercise duration, and intensity.

Set Baseline Measurements:

Establish baseline measurements for each chosen metric before starting your nutrition and exercise program. Record initial values using reliable measurement methods, such as body composition analysis, fitness assessments, and performance tests.

Use Tracking Tools:

Utilize tracking tools and resources to monitor your progress systematically. Consider using fitness apps, wearable devices, spreadsheets, or journals to record data consistently and track changes over time.

Monitor Nutritional Intake:

Track your daily nutritional intake by recording food and beverage consumption. Use food journals, nutrition apps, or online databases to log meals, snacks, portion sizes, macronutrient intake, and calorie consumption.

Keep Workout Logs:

Maintain detailed workout logs to track your exercise sessions and training progress. Record workout dates, exercise types, sets, repetitions, weights lifted, distances covered, durations, perceived exertion levels, and any relevant notes or observations.

Monitor Performance Indicators:

Monitor performance indicators during exercise to assess progress and adaptation. Pay attention to improvements in strength, endurance, speed, power, agility, flexibility, and recovery between workouts.

Assess Body Composition Changes:

Regularly assess changes in body composition to track changes in muscle mass, fat mass, and overall body composition. Use methods such as skinfold measurements, bioelectrical impedance analysis, DEXA scans, or waist-to-hip ratios.

Schedule Regular Assessments:

Schedule regular assessments at predetermined intervals to evaluate progress and adjust your nutrition and exercise plan accordingly. Aim for assessments every 4-6 weeks to allow sufficient time for meaningful changes to occur.

Analyze Trends and Patterns:

Analyze trends and patterns in your data to identify progress, plateaus, or regressions over time. Look for correlations between nutrition, exercise, lifestyle factors, and performance outcomes to inform your decision-making process.

Celebrate Milestones and Progress:

Celebrate milestones and achievements along the way, no matter how small. Acknowledge progress, improvements, and successes to stay motivated and reinforce positive behaviors.

Adjust Strategies as Needed:

Based on your assessment findings, adjust your nutrition and exercise strategies as needed to address areas of weakness, capitalize on strengths, and optimize your approach for continued progress and performance enhancement.

Making Adjustments to Nutrition and Exercise Plans Based on Results and Goals

Adjusting nutrition and exercise plans based on results and goals is a critical aspect of optimizing performance and achieving desired outcomes. By analyzing progress, identifying areas for improvement, and making informed adjustments, individuals can refine their strategies to better align with their goals and enhance overall performance. Here's a comprehensive guide to making adjustments to nutrition and exercise plans:

Review Your Goals:

Begin by revisiting your initial goals and objectives related to nutrition, exercise, and performance. Clarify your priorities, aspirations, and timelines to ensure alignment with your current aspirations and motivations.

135

Assess Your Progress:

Conduct a comprehensive assessment of your progress using relevant performance metrics, measurements, and data collected over time. Evaluate changes in body composition, strength, endurance, flexibility, and other key indicators of performance.

Identify Strengths and Weaknesses:

Identify strengths and weaknesses in your current nutrition and exercise plans based on your assessment findings. Recognize areas of success and areas that require improvement or adjustment to support your goals effectively.

Analyze Patterns and Trends:

Analyze patterns and trends in your data to identify recurring themes, correlations, and discrepancies. Look for factors influencing your progress, such as dietary habits, exercise routines, lifestyle factors, and external stressors.

Consider Lifestyle Factors:

Take into account lifestyle factors that may impact your ability to adhere to your nutrition and exercise plans. Consider factors such as work commitments, family responsibilities, social obligations, sleep patterns, and stress levels when making adjustments.

Consult with Professionals:

Seek guidance from qualified professionals, such as registered dietitians, sports nutritionists, personal trainers, and healthcare providers. Discuss your assessment findings, goals, and challenges to receive personalized recommendations and support.

Adjust Nutritional Intake:

Adjust your nutritional intake based on your goals, preferences, and assessment findings. Modify portion sizes, macronutrient ratios, meal timing, and food choices to better support your energy needs, performance goals, and overall well-being.

Modify Exercise Programming:

Modify your exercise programming to address areas of weakness and capitalize on strengths. Adjust workout intensity, volume, frequency, and exercise selection to stimulate adaptation, prevent plateaus, and promote continued progress.

Incorporate Variety and Progression:

Incorporate variety and progression into your nutrition and exercise plans to keep them engaging and effective. Experiment with new foods, recipes, training modalities, and workout formats to challenge your body and mind.

Set SMART Goals:

Set SMART (Specific, Measurable, Achievable, Relevant, Time-bound) goals to guide your adjustments and measure your progress effectively. Break larger goals into smaller, actionable steps to maintain focus and momentum.

Monitor and Reassess:

Continuously monitor your progress and reassess your nutrition and exercise plans to ensure they remain aligned with your evolving goals and priorities. Be open to making further adjustments as needed to optimize your approach over time.

Stay Flexible and Adaptive:

Stay flexible and adaptive in your approach to nutrition and exercise. Be willing to experiment, learn from setbacks, and adjust your plans based on feedback and experience.

CHAPTER 8

ACHIEVING SUSTAINABLE LONG-TERM PERFORMANCE

Sustainable long-term performance is the cornerstone of success in optimizing nutrition and exercise for peak performance. It involves adopting habits, routines, and strategies that promote consistency, resilience, and well-being over time. By prioritizing sustainability, individuals can achieve lasting results while maintaining a balanced and fulfilling lifestyle. Here's a comprehensive guide to achieving sustainable long-term performance:

Establish Clear Goals:

Begin by defining clear, achievable, and meaningful goals that align with your values, aspirations, and priorities. Set realistic expectations and establish a long-term vision for your health, fitness, and performance journey.

Focus on Behavior Change:

Shift your focus from short-term outcomes to sustainable behavior change. Emphasize the development of healthy habits, routines, and mindset shifts that support your long-term well-being and performance goals.

Cultivate Consistency:

Prioritize consistency in your nutrition and exercise practices by establishing regular habits and routines. Aim for gradual, sustainable progress over time rather than quick fixes or drastic changes that are difficult to maintain.

Embrace Variety and Enjoyment:

Embrace variety and enjoyment in your nutrition and exercise routines to keep them engaging and sustainable. Explore diverse foods, recipes, cuisines, and physical activities that align with your preferences and interests.

Practice Mindful Eating:

Cultivate mindfulness and awareness in your eating habits by paying attention to hunger cues, satiety signals, and food choices. Eat mindfully, savoring each bite, and honoring your body's nutritional needs without judgment or restriction.

Listen to Your Body:

Tune in to your body's signals and feedback to guide your nutrition and exercise decisions. Respect your body's limits, prioritize rest and recovery, and adjust your approach based on how you feel physically, mentally, and emotionally.

Prioritize Sleep and Stress Management:

Prioritize quality sleep and effective stress management as integral components of sustainable performance. Establish healthy sleep habits, manage stress levels, and practice relaxation techniques to support recovery, resilience, and overall well-being.

Foster Supportive Relationships:

Surround yourself with supportive individuals who uplift and encourage your journey towards optimal performance. Cultivate relationships with friends, family members, mentors, and peers who share your values and support your goals.

Adapt to Life Changes:

Stay flexible and adaptive in response to life changes, transitions, and challenges. Recognize that setbacks and obstacles are natural parts of the journey, and approach them with resilience, resourcefulness, and a growth mindset.

Practice Self-Compassion:

Be kind to yourself and practice self-compassion throughout your performance journey. Embrace imperfection, forgive setbacks, and treat yourself with the same kindness and understanding you would offer to a friend.

Monitor Progress and Adjustments:

Continuously monitor your progress, evaluate your strategies, and make adjustments as needed to support sustainable long-term performance. Stay engaged, proactive, and open to feedback from your experiences.

Celebrate Milestones and Progress:

Celebrate your achievements, milestones, and progress along the way. Acknowledge your hard work, dedication, and resilience, and take pride in the positive changes you've made towards optimizing your performance and well-being.

Emphasizing Consistency and Gradual Improvements

Consistency and gradual improvements are foundational principles in the pursuit of optimal performance through nutrition and exercise. By embracing these principles, individuals can establish sustainable habits, foster long-term progress, and ultimately achieve their performance goals. Here's how to emphasize consistency and gradual improvements in your journey toward peak performance:

Establish Sustainable Habits:

Focus on building sustainable habits that support your nutrition and exercise goals. Consistently prioritize behaviors that align with your values and aspirations, making them an integral part of your daily routine.

Prioritize Regularity Over Intensity:

Prioritize regularity and frequency in your nutrition and exercise routines over short bursts of intense effort. Consistent, moderate efforts over time yield greater benefits and are more sustainable in the long run.

Set Realistic Expectations:

Set realistic expectations for your progress and outcomes, understanding that meaningful changes take time and dedication. Avoid comparing yourself to others and focus on your personal journey of growth and improvement.

Celebrate Small Victories:

Celebrate small victories and achievements along the way, no matter how insignificant they may seem. Recognize and appreciate the progress you make, reinforcing positive behaviors and motivating continued effort.

Embrace the Process:

Embrace the process of growth and development, recognizing that sustainable change is a journey rather than a destination. Enjoy the journey, learn from your experiences, and trust in your ability to evolve over time.

Focus on Long-Term Sustainability:

Prioritize long-term sustainability over short-term gains or quick fixes. Choose nutrition and exercise strategies that you can maintain consistently over time, integrating them seamlessly into your lifestyle.

Practice Patience and Persistence:

Practice patience and persistence in your pursuit of optimal performance. Understand that progress may be gradual and nonlinear, requiring perseverance and resilience in the face of setbacks and challenges.

Track Progress and Reflect Regularly:

Track your progress and reflect regularly on your nutrition and exercise practices. Keep a journal, use tracking tools, and periodically assess your habits, behaviors, and outcomes to identify areas for improvement.

Adjust and Adapt:

Be flexible and willing to adjust your approach based on feedback and results. Continuously refine your nutrition and exercise strategies, making incremental adjustments to better align with your evolving needs and goals.

Prioritize Consistency Over Perfection:

Prioritize consistency over perfection in your nutrition and exercise efforts. Focus on making small, sustainable changes that accumulate over time, rather than striving for an unattainable standard of perfection.

Cultivate a Growth Mindset:

Cultivate a growth mindset that embraces challenges, learns from failures, and sees setbacks as opportunities for learning and growth. Approach each day with curiosity, resilience, and a willingness to improve.

Developing a Supportive Environment and Social Network

Creating a supportive environment and cultivating a strong social network are integral components of achieving optimal performance through nutrition and exercise. A positive support system can provide encouragement, accountability, and motivation, making the journey towards peak performance more enjoyable and sustainable. Here's how to develop a supportive environment and social network to enhance your nutrition and exercise practices:

Identify Supportive Individuals:

Identify individuals in your life who share your values and goals related to nutrition and exercise. Seek out friends, family members, colleagues, and peers who can offer encouragement, understanding, and support along your journey.

Communicate Your Goals:

Communicate your goals, aspirations, and challenges openly and honestly with your support network. Share your vision for optimal performance and invite others to join you on your journey, fostering a sense of camaraderie and mutual accountability.

Surround Yourself with Positive Influences:

Surround yourself with positive influences and role models who inspire and uplift you in your pursuit of peak performance. Seek out individuals who embody the values and behaviors you aspire to emulate, drawing inspiration from their successes and achievements.

Participate in Group Activities:

Participate in group activities, classes, or clubs related to nutrition and exercise that foster a sense of community and belonging. Join fitness groups, sports teams, or recreational leagues where you can connect with like-minded individuals and share common interests.

Foster Supportive Relationships:

Cultivate supportive relationships based on trust, respect, and empathy. Be there for others in your support network, offering encouragement, listening ear, and practical assistance when needed. Foster a culture of mutual support and reciprocity within your social circle.

Attend Workshops and Events:

Attend workshops, seminars, and events focused on nutrition, exercise, and performance optimization. Engage with experts, professionals, and enthusiasts in the field, expanding your knowledge, skills, and network of contacts.

Seek Professional Guidance:

Seek guidance from qualified professionals, such as registered dietitians, personal trainers, and sports psychologists, who can provide expert advice and support tailored to your individual needs and goals. Build collaborative relationships with professionals who understand your aspirations and can help you navigate challenges along the way.

Create Shared Experiences:

Create opportunities for shared experiences and bonding within your social network. Organize group workouts, outdoor adventures, cooking classes, or wellness retreats where you can connect with others while pursuing health and fitness goals together.

Utilize Online Communities and Resources:

Tap into online communities, forums, and social media platforms dedicated to nutrition, exercise, and performance enhancement. Connect with individuals from diverse backgrounds and experiences, sharing insights, tips, and encouragement in a supportive virtual environment.

Practice Active Listening and Empathy:

Practice active listening and empathy when engaging with members of your support network. Validate their experiences, acknowledge their efforts, and offer constructive feedback and encouragement in return.

Celebrate Successes Together:

Celebrate successes, milestones, and achievements within your support network, recognizing the collective progress and accomplishments of each member. Share victories, big and small, and acknowledge the contributions of everyone towards the common goal of optimal performance.

Strategies for Preventing Burnout and Injury

Preventing burnout and injury is crucial for maintaining optimal performance and overall well-being in nutrition and exercise routines. Incorporating strategies to prevent burnout and injury helps individuals sustain long-term progress and enjoyment in their fitness journey. Here are effective strategies for preventing burnout and injury:

Gradual Progression:

Emphasize gradual progression in your exercise routines, gradually increasing intensity, duration, or frequency over time. Avoid sudden spikes in training volume or intensity that may increase the risk of overuse injuries and burnout.

Proper Warm-Up and Cool-Down:

Prioritize a thorough warm-up before exercise to prepare your body for activity, increase blood flow to muscles, and improve flexibility and range of motion. Incorporate dynamic stretches, mobility drills, and light cardio to prime your body for movement. Similarly, include a cooldown routine to aid in recovery and reduce muscle soreness post-workout.

Listen to Your Body:

Tune in to your body's signals and respond accordingly to prevent overtraining and injury. Pay attention to signs of fatigue, pain, discomfort, or decreased performance, and adjust your workout intensity, duration, or type as needed.

Rest and Recovery:

Prioritize adequate rest and recovery periods between workouts to allow your body to repair, regenerate, and adapt to training stimuli. Incorporate active recovery activities such as walking, yoga, or swimming on rest days to promote circulation and reduce muscle stiffness.

Periodization:

Implement a periodized training program that incorporates planned cycles of varying intensity, volume, and recovery to prevent overtraining and optimize performance. Periodization allows for structured progression while minimizing the risk of burnout and injury.

Cross-Training:

Incorporate cross-training activities into your fitness routine to prevent overuse injuries and maintain overall balance and functionality. Include a variety of exercises, sports, and recreational activities that target different muscle groups and movement patterns.

Proper Technique and Form:

Prioritize proper technique and form during exercise to reduce the risk of injury and maximize performance gains. Focus on quality movement patterns, maintain neutral alignment, and avoid compensatory movements or excessive joint stress.

Recovery Strategies:

Implement effective recovery strategies such as foam rolling, massage therapy, compression garments, and contrast baths to alleviate muscle soreness, reduce inflammation, and enhance recovery between workouts.

Nutritional Support:

Ensure proper nutrition and hydration to support recovery, repair, and adaptation processes following exercise. Consume a balanced diet rich in nutrient-dense foods, hydrate adequately, and replenish electrolytes lost through sweat during intense workouts.

Sleep Hygiene:

Prioritize quality sleep and establish healthy sleep hygiene practices to support recovery, hormone regulation, and overall well-being. Aim for 7-9 hours of uninterrupted sleep per night, create a relaxing bedtime routine, and create a comfortable sleep environment free of distractions.

Manage Stress:

Implement stress management techniques such as mindfulness meditation, deep breathing exercises, yoga, or progressive muscle relaxation to reduce stress levels and promote relaxation and recovery.

Listen to Professional Advice:

Seek guidance from qualified professionals such as certified personal trainers, physical therapists, and sports medicine specialists for personalized recommendations and support in injury prevention and recovery.

Celebrating Achievements and Maintaining Motivation

Celebrating achievements and maintaining motivation are essential components of sustaining progress and enthusiasm in your journey towards optimal performance through nutrition and exercise. By acknowledging successes, both big and small, and cultivating intrinsic motivation, individuals can stay committed, inspired, and empowered to pursue their performance goals. Here are effective strategies for celebrating achievements and maintaining motivation:

Set Meaningful Milestones:

Establish meaningful milestones and benchmarks along your performance journey. Break down larger goals into smaller, attainable targets that you can celebrate as you progress, providing a sense of accomplishment and momentum.

Reflect on Progress:

Take time to reflect on your progress and achievements regularly. Celebrate the milestones you've reached, recognize the improvements you've made, and acknowledge the efforts and dedication you've invested in your nutrition and exercise routines.

Practice Gratitude:

Cultivate an attitude of gratitude for the progress and opportunities that come your way. Express appreciation for the support of others, the resources available to you, and the experiences that enrich your journey towards peak performance.

Reward Yourself:

Reward yourself for reaching milestones and achieving goals with meaningful incentives or rewards. Treat yourself to a special meal, indulge in a relaxing spa day, or invest in new fitness gear as a token of recognition for your hard work and dedication.

Share Your Achievements:

Share your achievements and successes with your support network, whether it's friends, family, or fellow enthusiasts. Celebrate your progress together, inspire others with your accomplishments, and bask in the encouragement and validation of your peers.

Visualize Success:

Visualize your success and imagine yourself achieving your performance goals with clarity and conviction. Use visualization techniques to create mental images of your desired outcomes, reinforcing your motivation and commitment to your aspirations.

Keep a Success Journal:

Keep a success journal to document your achievements, breakthroughs, and moments of triumph. Write down your proudest moments, reflect on the challenges you've overcome, and revisit your accomplishments whenever you need a boost of motivation.

Stay Inspired:

Seek inspiration from role models, mentors, and individuals who embody the qualities and achievements you aspire to attain. Surround yourself with positive influences, motivational quotes, and uplifting stories that fuel your determination and drive.

Find Joy in the Process:

Find joy and fulfillment in the process of pursuing your nutrition and exercise goals, rather than solely focusing on the end results. Embrace the journey, savor the moments of growth and discovery, and celebrate the resilience and determination that define your pursuit of peak performance.

Stay Flexible and Adaptive:

Stay flexible and adaptive in your approach to achieving optimal performance. Embrace challenges, learn from setbacks, and adjust your strategies as needed to stay aligned with your evolving aspirations and priorities.

Cultivate Intrinsic Motivation:

Cultivate intrinsic motivation by connecting with your personal values, passions, and aspirations. Align your goals with what truly matters to you, tap into your inner drive and purpose, and find fulfillment in the pursuit of excellence for its own sake.

Celebrate Every Step Forward:

Celebrate every step forward, no matter how small or incremental it may seem. Acknowledge the progress you've made, honor the effort you've invested, and recognize the resilience and determination that propel you towards your peak performance goals.

CHAPTER 8

CONCLUSION

In the journey towards optimal performance, mastering the intricate interplay between nutrition and exercise is key to unlocking your full potential. "How to Fuel Your Body for Optimal Performance: A Comprehensive Guide to Nutrition and Exercise for Peak Performance" has been a comprehensive roadmap, guiding you through the principles, strategies, and practices essential for achieving peak performance and vitality.

Throughout this guide, we've explored the fundamental importance of nutrition and exercise in enhancing physical and mental well-being, optimizing performance, and supporting overall health. From understanding the synergy between nutrition and exercise to designing personalized nutrition plans and exercise routines, each chapter has equipped you with actionable insights and practical tools to fuel your body for success.

We've delved into the significance of consistency, gradual improvements, and sustainable habits in maintaining long-term progress and preventing burnout and injury. By prioritizing self-care, listening to your body, and fostering a supportive environment, you've learned how to navigate challenges, celebrate achievements, and stay motivated on your performance journey.

As you conclude this guide, remember that achieving optimal performance is not a destination but a continuous journey of growth, discovery, and self-mastery. Embrace the process, honor the setbacks, and celebrate the victories, knowing that every step forward brings you closer to realizing your full potential.

Whether you're an athlete striving for excellence, a fitness enthusiast pursuing personal goals, or simply someone committed to living a healthier, more vibrant life, the principles outlined in this book are applicable to all who seek to optimize their performance and well-being.

As you apply the knowledge and insights gained from "How to Fuel Your Body for

Optimal Performance," may you embark on your journey with confidence, resilience, and a deep sense of purpose. Remember that the power to fuel your body, transform your performance, and live your best life lies within you.

Here's to embracing the journey, pursuing your passions, and unleashing the boundless potential that resides within you. May your commitment to optimal nutrition, exercise, and peak performance be a testament to the extraordinary heights you can achieve when you nourish your body, mind, and spirit with intention and purpose.

Recap of Key Principles and Strategies for Optimal Performance

Throughout "How to Fuel Your Body for Optimal Performance: A Comprehensive Guide to Nutrition and Exercise for Peak Performance," we have explored a myriad of principles and strategies essential for unlocking your full potential and achieving peak performance. As we recap, let's revisit the key principles and strategies highlighted in this comprehensive guide:

Understanding Optimal Performance:

Optimal performance is the culmination of balanced nutrition, tailored exercise, and holistic well-being. It encompasses physical, mental, and emotional aspects of health and vitality.

Synergy Between Nutrition and Exercise:

Nutrition and exercise are synergistic components that work hand in hand to optimize performance. By aligning your nutrition with your exercise regimen, you can enhance energy levels, promote recovery, and maximize performance gains.

Consistency and Gradual Improvements:

Consistency and gradual improvements form the cornerstone of sustainable progress. By prioritizing regularity over intensity and celebrating incremental achievements, you can maintain momentum and prevent burnout.

Personalized Nutrition Plans:

Designing personalized nutrition plans involves assessing individual needs, preferences, and goals. By incorporating balanced meals, mindful eating practices, and strategic nutrient timing, you can fuel your body effectively for optimal performance.

Exercise Programming for Peak Performance:

Exercise programming for peak performance requires a balanced approach that targets strength, endurance, flexibility, and agility. By incorporating diverse exercises, periodization techniques, and proper recovery strategies, you can optimize your physical capabilities.

Integrating Nutrition and Exercise:

Integrating nutrition and exercise involves aligning dietary choices with workout sessions to optimize performance and recovery. By timing meals and snacks strategically and choosing optimal foods for pre- and post-workout fueling, you can support your body's needs throughout the training process.

Preventing Burnout and Injury:

Preventing burnout and injury is paramount for sustaining long-term progress and well-being. By prioritizing rest and recovery, practicing proper technique and form, and listening to your body's signals, you can minimize the risk of overuse injuries and mental fatigue.

Celebrating Achievements and Maintaining Motivation:

Celebrating achievements and maintaining motivation are vital for sustaining enthusiasm and commitment. By setting meaningful milestones, practicing gratitude, and sharing successes with your support network, you can stay inspired and focused on your performance goals.

Encouragement for Continued Dedication to Nutrition and Exercise

As you reach the conclusion of "How to Fuel Your Body for Optimal Performance: A Comprehensive Guide to Nutrition and Exercise for Peak Performance," it's important to recognize the journey you've embarked upon and the commitment you've shown towards optimizing your performance and well-being. Your dedication to embracing the principles of nutrition and exercise for peak performance is commendable, and it's vital to stay motivated and inspired as you continue on your path.

In the pursuit of optimal performance, it's natural to encounter challenges, setbacks, and moments of doubt. However, it's during these times that your resilience, determination, and unwavering commitment to your goals truly shine. Remember that every step forward, no matter how small, brings you closer to realizing your full potential and living the vibrant, fulfilling life you deserve.

As you navigate your journey, I encourage you to hold onto the following principles and reminders:

Believe in Yourself: Trust in your abilities, your potential, and your capacity to achieve greatness. Cultivate a mindset of self-belief and confidence, knowing that you have the strength and resilience to overcome any obstacle in your path.

Stay Consistent: Consistency is the cornerstone of progress and success. Commit to showing up for yourself each day, honoring your nutrition and exercise routines, and making choices that align with your goals and values.

Celebrate Progress: Take time to celebrate every milestone, achievement, and victory along the way. Acknowledge the progress you've made, no matter how small, and let each success fuel your motivation and determination to keep pushing forward.

Embrace the Journey: Embrace the journey of self-discovery, growth, and transformation. Embrace the highs and the lows, the triumphs and the challenges, knowing that each experience holds valuable lessons and opportunities for growth.

Find Joy in Movement:

Rediscover the joy and exhilaration that comes from movement and physical activity. Explore new forms of exercise, challenge yourself to try new activities, and find what brings you true happiness and fulfillment in your fitness journey.

Nourish Your Body and Mind:

Prioritize nourishing your body with wholesome, nutrient-dense foods and nurturing your mind with positive thoughts and self-care practices. Remember that optimal performance encompasses not just physical strength, but also mental resilience and emotional well-being.

Seek Support:

Surround yourself with a supportive community of friends, family, mentors, and peers who uplift and encourage you on your journey. Lean on them for guidance, motivation, and accountability, knowing that you are never alone in your pursuit of greatness.

Be Kind to Yourself: Practice self-compassion, forgiveness, and kindness towards yourself. Treat setbacks and challenges as opportunities for growth and learning, and remember that self-care is an essential part of the journey towards optimal performance.

Stay Curious and Open-Minded: Approach your nutrition and exercise journey with curiosity, openness, and a willingness to learn. Stay receptive to new ideas, perspectives, and strategies that may enhance your performance and well-being.

Never Give Up: Above all, never give up on yourself or your dreams. Stay resilient, determined, and steadfast in your commitment to becoming the best version of yourself, knowing that the journey towards optimal performance is one of endless possibilities and opportunities.

As you continue your dedication to nutrition and exercise, may you find inspiration, fulfillment, and joy in every step of the journey. Remember that the pursuit of optimal performance is not just about reaching a destination it's about embracing the process, savoring the moments, and living each day with purpose and passion.

With dedication, perseverance, and a steadfast commitment to your goals, you have the power to transform your life, elevate your performance, and achieve greatness beyond measure. Keep moving forward, keep striving for excellence, and never underestimate the incredible potential that lies within you.

Final Thoughts on the Journey Toward Peak Performance

As we come to the culmination of "How to Fuel Your Body for Optimal Performance: A Comprehensive Guide to Nutrition and Exercise for Peak Performance," it's essential to reflect on the profound journey you've undertaken. Your exploration of nutrition, exercise, and their symbiotic

173

relationship in enhancing performance has been a testament to your dedication, curiosity, and commitment to living your best life.

The journey toward peak performance is not merely about reaching a destination; it's about embracing the process, discovering your strengths, and uncovering the depths of your potential along the way. Throughout this guide, you've delved into the intricacies of fueling your body, optimizing your routines, and cultivating the mindset necessary for sustainable success.

As you reflect on your journey toward peak performance, consider these final thoughts:

It's a Holistic Journey: Peak performance encompasses more than just physical prowess it's a holistic journey that integrates nutrition, exercise, mindset, and lifestyle choices. Embrace the interconnectedness of these elements and strive for balance, harmony, and alignment in all aspects of your life.

Embrace the Growth Mindset: Adopt a growth mindset that celebrates challenges, learns from setbacks, and thrives on continuous improvement. Embrace the process of growth, knowing that every obstacle is an opportunity for learning, resilience, and personal evolution.

Celebrate Your Progress: Take a moment to celebrate how far you've come on your journey. Acknowledge the progress you've made, the obstacles you've overcome, and the lessons you've learned along the way. Celebrate not just the destination but also the milestones, both big and small, that mark your path to greatness.

Stay True to Your Values: Remember the values and principles that guide your journey toward peak performance. Stay true to your authentic self, honor your core beliefs, and let your actions reflect the integrity, passion, and purpose that define your pursuit of excellence.

175

Keep Exploring and Evolving: Peak performance is a dynamic, ever-evolving process. Keep exploring new possibilities, experimenting with different strategies, and pushing the boundaries of your comfort zone. Embrace change, adapt to challenges, and welcome the opportunity for growth and expansion in every aspect of your life.

Share Your Wisdom: Share your wisdom, insights, and experiences with others who may be embarking on their own journey toward peak performance. Pay it forward, inspire others, and be a guiding light for those who seek guidance, support, and encouragement along the way.

Trust the Journey: Trust in the journey and have faith in your ability to overcome obstacles and achieve your goals. Trust in the resilience of the human spirit, the power of perseverance, and the transformative potential that lies within you.

Gratitude Is Key: Cultivate an attitude of gratitude for the opportunities, experiences, and relationships that enrich your life. Take a moment to express gratitude for the support of others, the lessons learned from challenges, and the blessings that surround you each day.

Your Potential Is Limitless:

Remember that your potential for greatness is limitless. Believe in yourself, dream big, and never underestimate the extraordinary capabilities that reside within you. With dedication, determination, and a steadfast commitment to your goals, anything is possible.

The Journey Continues: As you

conclude this guide, remember that the journey toward peak performance is an ongoing adventure one that unfolds with each step you take, each choice you make, and each moment you embrace with intention and purpose. Embrace the journey, cherish the moments, and let the pursuit of peak performance be a lifelong quest for excellence, vitality, and fulfillment.

9 798888 340587 6